IT HAPPENED TO ME

Series Editor: Arlene Hirschfelder

Books in the "It Happened to Me" series are designed for inquisitive teens digging for answers about certain illnesses, social issues, or lifestyle interests. Whether you are deep into your teen years or just entering them, these books are gold mines of up-to-date information, riveting teen views, and great visuals to help you figure out stuff. Besides special boxes highlighting singular facts, each book is enhanced with the latest reading lists, websites, and an index. Perfect for browsing, there's loads of expert information by acclaimed writers to help parents, guardians, and librarians understand teen illness, tough situations, and lifestyle choices.

1. *Learning Disabilities: The Ultimate Teen Guide,* by Penny Hutchins Paquette and Cheryl Gerson Tuttle, 2003.
2. *Epilepsy: The Ultimate Teen Guide,* by Kathlyn Gay and Sean McGarrahan, 2002.
3. *Stress Relief: The Ultimate Teen Guide,* by Mark Powell, 2002.
4. *Making Sexual Decisions: The Ultimate Teen Guide,* by L. Kris Gowen, Ph.D., 2003.
5. *Asthma: The Ultimate Teen Guide,* by Penny Hutchins Paquette, 2003.
6. *Cultural Diversity: Conflicts and Challenges: The Ultimate Teen Guide,* by Kathlyn Gay, 2003.
7. *Diabetes: The Ultimate Teen Guide,* by Katherine J. Moran, 2004.
8. *When Will I Stop Hurting?: Teens, Loss, and Grief: The Ultimate Teen Guide,* by Edward Myers, 2004.

Diabetes

The Ultimate Teen Guide

KATHERINE J. MORAN, MSN, RN, CDE

**Illustrations by
Lisa P. Merriman**

It Happened to Me, No. 7

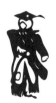

The Scarecrow Press, Inc.
Lanham, Maryland • Toronto • Oxford
2004

SCARECROW PRESS, INC.

Published in the United States of America
by Scarecrow Press, Inc.
A wholly owned subsidary of The Rowman & Littlefield Publishing Group, Inc.
4501 Forbes Boulevard, Suite 200, Lanham, Maryland 20706
www.scarecrowpress.com

PO Box 317
Oxford
OX2 9RU, UK

British Library Cataloguing in Publication Information Available

Library of Congress Cataloging-in-Publication Data

Moran, Katherine J., 1959–
  Diabetes : the ultimate teen guide / Katherine J. Moran ; illustrations by Lisa P.
Merriman.
    p. cm. – (It happened to me ; no. 7)
  Summary: Provides practical information on living with diabetes, discussing
what the disease is, how to manage it, treatment options, and related issuess.
  Includes bibliographical references and index.
  ISBN 0-8108-4806-6
1.   Diabetes in children—Juvenile literature. 2. Diabetes in adolescence—
Juvenile literature. 3. Consumer education. [1. Diabetes. 2. Diseases.] I.
Merriman, Lisa P., ill. II. Title. III. Series.
RJ420.D5 M67 2004
616.4'62–dc22
                                                                2003018500

In dedication to my family and friends . . .
you have all *helped* me more than you will ever know.
In tribute to my daughter Nicole . . .
you have *taught* me more than you will ever know.
My love to you all.

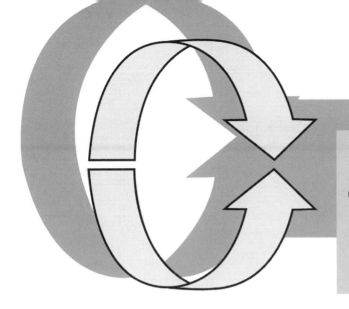

Contents

Contents

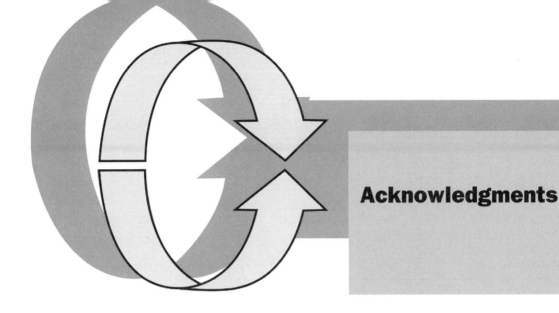

Acknowledgments

I would like to acknowledge those who assisted me in the completion of this project: my sister, Lisa Merriman, for sharing her wonderful illustrations—she is truly a gifted artist; LuRee Buchmann, R.N.C., B.S.N., M.S.A., M.Ed., my mentor, for her support, direction, and editing expertise; Judy Nechal, B.S.N., R.N., C.D.E. and Marilyn Anderson, R.D., C.D.E. for reviewing the book and offering their expert opinions; and finally, Pelleassa Brock for her guidance and support in addressing the technical issues of the book.

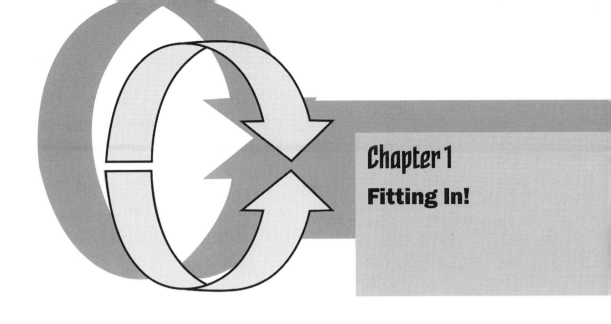

Chapter 1
Fitting In!

Yesterday the biggest problem you had was that huge (not really) zit on the side of your nose. Today you're probably thinking this diabetes is just another cruel life joke. Right? You've gone from trying to determine who you are, and why you are who you are, to dealing with diabetes. Can it get any worse?

Well, as they say, hang in there. It's always darkest before the dawn. Okay, so now you're probably thinking, "What in the heck does that mean?!" Well, it doesn't mean that just like the pimple eventually went away, this will too. But, you certainly can and will have a full life. Just remember one thing: You, like everyone else, are a unique individual who just happens to have diabetes. Yes, your good health will require extra attention, and yes it's a pain in the butt, but it will pay off in the end (no pun intended!). Don't believe me? Take a look at people with diabetes who consistently go through all that management stuff. You know the drill: checking blood glucose, taking insulin, exercising, counting carbohydrates (a.k.a., carbs), and so on. Well, they statistically have less complications; it's a proven fact. Not good enough? Okay, how about this, *you will feel better*! Running to the bathroom every five minutes is not anyone's idea of a good time, and neither is having a blood sugar so low that you can't get your mouth to work—not to mention the fact that after you recover (if you can call it that) you feel like you got hit by a freaking truck! Yeah, management is a pain, but it's worth it.

Another thing to keep in mind, your diabetes isn't like the zit on your nose. No one can see it. It's up to you to decide whom you choose to share this part of *you* with. Life is like that. You really have a lot of choices. And that doesn't just mean who knows about your diabetes, but about a lot of other things too . . . more about that later.

Life is what you make it. . . . So, go out and make it good!

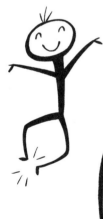

You have control over the path you take in your life! —Nicole Johnson, Miss America, 1999

You're a shining star! —Gary Hall Jr., Olympic Gold medalist, 1996 and 2000

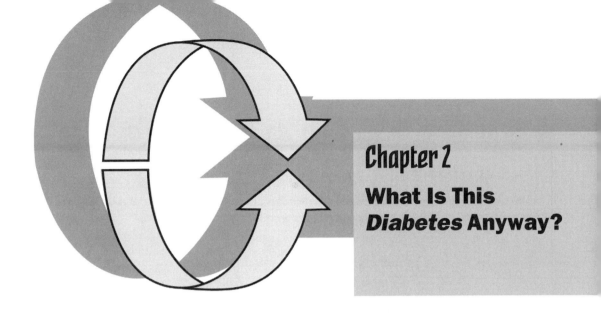

Chapter 2
What Is This *Diabetes* Anyway?

There are several kinds of diabetes. But the two major types of diabetes that we are going to focus on are type 1 and type 2. The type of diabetes usually seen in children and young adults is type 1 diabetes (known for years as insulin-dependent diabetes mellitus or juvenile diabetes), whereas the type of diabetes usually seen in adults is type 2 diabetes (previously known as adult onset diabetes or noninsulin-dependent diabetes mellitus).

But, before we begin talking about what happens in the body when diabetes occurs, let's talk about what normally happens in the body as it relates to metabolism (cellular use of glucose for energy). For example, let's talk about what happens in a person who *does not* have diabetes. That way it will be clearer when we talk about what happens when a person *does* have diabetes.

Okay, let's start with the digestion of food. You remember this right? When you eat (just about everything and anything), your body actually starts to break down the food in your mouth with the help of your saliva (yes, it actually has a purpose). Then, when you swallow the food and it reaches your stomach, more digestion takes place. This process continues until eventually the food reaches your intestines (the small intestines first), where it is absorbed through the walls of the intestines as glucose (a form of sugar the body can use for energy), enters the bloodstream, and is transported by the bloodstream to all the cells of your body. But, when the glucose in the blood reaches the pancreas (a gland located behind your stomach), the beta cells (located in the tail of the pancreas) are stimulated to make the hormone insulin. The insulin pairs up with the glucose

STRANGE BUT TRUE

1500 B.C. Diabetes was first described in ancient Egypt. Early healers noticed that ants were attracted to the urine of people with diabetes because of the sugar.[1]

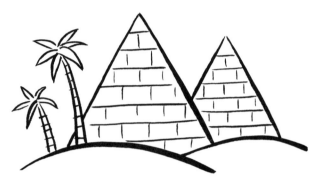

100 A.D. A Greek physician calls the disease diabetes, meaning *siphon*, because people with diabetes urinate so often.[2]

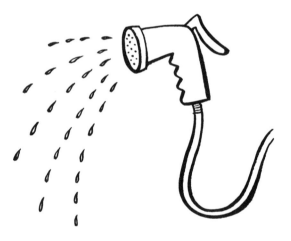

(continued)

that's in the blood, goes to all the cells in the body, and helps the glucose get into the cells (where it can be used for energy).

So, what happens when a person develops diabetes? Well, either the body is no longer making insulin (type 1 diabetes) or the insulin that is available doesn't work very well (type 2 diabetes). Either way, the result is the same; the glucose in the blood can't get into the cells. Consequently, the glucose stays in the bloodstream, causing damage to body organs.

STRANGE BUT TRUE

1000 Greek physicians order exercise on horseback to relieve the symptoms of diabetes.[3]

1869 Paul Langerhans discovers islet cells in the pancreas.[4]

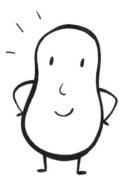

1889 Scientists discover that removing the pancreas from dogs causes diabetes.[5]

1921 Canadian scientists Dr. Banting and Dr. Best give insulin to a boy with diabetes. He lives until adulthood.[6]

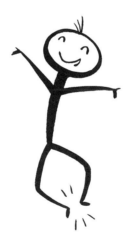

(continued)

WHAT CAUSES DIABETES?

Diabetes develops in people who have family genes that predispose them to develop diabetes when they are exposed to environmental triggers. So, "What does that mean?" Well, there are many theories, but one theory that some scientists believe happens in type 1 diabetes is that the body is exposed to a virus that looks very

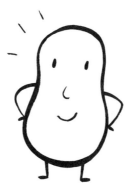
similar to the body's own beta cells. As you know, when viruses, bacteria, or anything foreign invades your body, it makes antibodies against the foreign substance, surrounds it, and finally kills it. Well, in the case of type 1 diabetes, when the body makes antibodies in response to the invading virus and starts to fight it off, the body mistakes the beta cells as the invading virus (because they look so much alike) and kills them off as well. So, when the body gets rid of the virus, it gets screwed up a little bit and gets rid of some of the body's own beta cells at the same time. This causes the person to have what is known as a *complete lack* of insulin (he or she no longer has the ability to make insulin because the beta cells are gone) and he or she develops type 1 diabetes.

In type 2 diabetes the environmental trigger is a little different and so is the body's response. There is still a genetic component to type 2 diabetes; in fact, it seems to be even stronger than in type 1 diabetes. However, the environmental triggers include things like being overweight and being inactive (old couch potato syndrome). For some reason, when a person has the genetic background to develop diabetes and he or she is overweight or inactive, the body's cells start to develop an attitude! This is known as insulin resistance. When this happens, the cells don't recognize insulin as being *insulin* anymore. As a result, the cells won't allow the insulin to do its job. So you see, the result is the same. Glucose can't get into the cells to be used for energy.

Remember, insulin is real important because its job is to pair up with glucose (sugar) in the bloodstream, go to all of the body cells, and then help the glucose get into the cells. When insulin reaches the cells it acts like a key and opens the doors on the body's cells to let the glucose in.[7] Without insulin, the glucose in the blood can't get into the cell where it is supposed to be burned for energy. Instead, the glucose stays in the blood and, if left untreated, begins to damage the body's organs. That's why all people with type 1 diabetes have to take at least one shot of insulin every day.

Speaking of glucose, there are a couple of places the body can get glucose to use for energy. For example, the body can get glucose from what you eat (and that includes anything you eat, not just food with sugar in it), and it can also get glucose from what the liver makes. The body can actually produce glucose in the liver, or it can release stored glucose from the liver and muscle.[8] The glucose from the liver is released into the blood stream whenever needed, like when you're sleeping and haven't eaten for a while. That way your cells have something to use for energy until you eat again! A person without diabetes makes enough insulin to help both sources of glucose enter the body's cells. Diabetes, however, interferes with this process. Let's talk about what happens.

WHAT HAPPENS WHEN A PERSON DEVELOPS DIABETES?

Your body is kinda like a car (bear with me here). It constantly needs energy for all body functions. For example, a car needs gas (sugar/food) to burn for energy, right? Okay, so when you want to go for a ride, what do you have to do first? Put gas in your car! You go to the gas station and use the gas nozzle (the insulin) to put the gas (food) into your car (your body—follow me?). Without the gas nozzle you can't get the gas into your car and without gas, your car won't go!

See, it all makes sense. When a person has type 1 diabetes the pancreas doesn't make insulin anymore, and when a person has type 2 diabetes, even though he or she has insulin, it just doesn't work. Either way, the glucose in the bloodstream doesn't have any way of getting into the body's cells to be burned for energy. But wait, that's not all that insulin does. Insulin also shuts off the body's production of glucose by the liver.[9] When insulin levels are too low, the liver makes too much glucose (remember what we said happens at night when you're sleeping) because there's nothing to shut it off. That means the blood glucose level continues to rise (because the glucose can't get into the cells). When it reaches a high level, the glucose begins to spill over into the urine.

See, that's the body's way of trying to stay in balance. It tries to get rid of the extra glucose in the blood through the formation of

When my blood glucose is high—I am very thirsty.
—Everett

urine. This is how it works: When the amount of glucose in the blood exceeds a certain point (usually around 160 mg/dl), the body pulls water from cells to help flush the extra glucose through the urine. That's why you spend so much time in the bathroom! Some of the other symptoms you may *experience* include:

1. *Thirst* (*really* thirsty!)—because you're urinating a lot, you get very thirsty!

2. *Hunger*—because the body's cells aren't getting any glucose, they're hungry.

3. *Tiredness*—when your cells can't get energy they get tired, and so do you!

4. *Weight loss*—when the body can't use glucose for energy, it starts to burn fat and protein for energy, which causes rapid weight loss.

5. *Ketones in the urine*—(seen mostly in people with type 1 diabetes) when the body burns fat for energy, the byproducts of fat breakdown are ketones. These ketones can become a problem if the body can't get rid of them. For example, if the blood glucose is high enough for long enough, ketones can build up in the blood and spill over into the urine.

6. *Ketoacidosis*—ketones are actually a form of acid that can make you very sick very quickly if your body can't get rid of them fast enough. Symptoms of ketoacidosis (ketone build up in the blood) may include an upset stomach, vomiting, or even a fruity smell to your breath (we'll talk more about this later).

WHAT HAPPENS WHEN A PERSON DEVELOPS DIABETES?

So, we know that people with type 1 diabetes will need insulin injections for the rest of their lives. However, initially some people experience what's known as a honeymoon (no . . . it's not what you think!). The honeymoon phase is more like a grace period that occurs a short time after the onset of the diabetes.[10] It usually starts within a couple weeks or so. During the honeymoon phase there is just enough insulin being made to allow some glucose to enter the cells. The honeymoon period may last a few weeks, a few months, or even a few years.

During this time the body may only need small amounts of insulin. After this period, however, the body will again need more exogenous (from injection) insulin. If you are one of those people that experienced the honeymoon phase, it is extremely important for you to remember one thing: Once you develop type 1 diabetes you will *always* need to take insulin. If you don't take your insulin your blood glucose will continue to rise and you will become *very* ill. Even though you have to take insulin, remember the only difference between you and someone without diabetes is that your body doesn't make enough insulin. That's it!

WHAT IS TYPE 2 DIABETES?

Now let's talk more about type 2 diabetes. Most of the time type 2 diabetes is found in adults (that's why it used to be called adult onset diabetes), but sometimes type 2 diabetes develops in teenagers or even children who are overweight. The major difference between type 1 and type 2 diabetes is that in type 2 diabetes insulin is still being made; it just doesn't work very well. Even though insulin is being made, when it gets to the cells the cells are moody (a cell with an attitude!!) and don't allow the insulin to do its job. That's because the body cells don't recognize the insulin as the *key*, and we know that extra fat cells in the body make the situation worse. Unfortunately, there has been an increase in the number of obese children and teens in the United States over the past few years.[11] That could also be the reason why there's been an increase of type 2 diabetes among adolescents as well. See, our population keeps getting larger and larger! You may be thinking, "Why is that?" Well, part of the problem may be due to genes (basic parts of heredity), but certainly part of the problem is also due to inactivity and overeating. How many times have you heard, "Would you like to *supersize* your meal for 39 cents?" When you think about it, it's not such a good deal after all! Anyway, that's why meal planning and physical activity really work well to treat this type of diabetes. Remember, the problem with type 2 diabetes is that the cells of the body become resistant to insulin.

Sometimes though, meal planning and physical activity aren't enough either. That's when people with this type of diabetes have to start taking pills to help control their blood glucose levels. These pills are not insulin, though. Insulin is a protein (kind of like the protein in meat) and is broken down by enzymes (acid) in the stomach, so it can't be taken in pill form. The pills people take for type 2 diabetes either help the pancreas make more insulin, help the person's cells become more sensitive to insulin, or even slow down the absorption of glucose through the gut. These pills can't help people with type 1 diabetes make more insulin because the beta cells in their pancreases are no longer functioning.

Sometimes, though, even the person with type 2 diabetes must take insulin injections. That doesn't mean that he or she now has type 1 diabetes. It just means that this person needs insulin injections to bring his or her blood glucose down to a healthy level. The person with type 2 diabetes uses insulin to help the body's insulin that's already there, but having trouble working.

CAN MY DIABETES CHANGE?

If you have type 1 diabetes you may be wondering if it will turn into type 2 diabetes as you grow older. Or, if you have type 2 diabetes if it will turn into type 1 diabetes. The answer is no. People with type 1 diabetes will always have type 1, and people with type 2 will always have type 2 diabetes. The two conditions are different. Type 1 and type 2 diabetes are inherited differently and have different reasons for causing the blood glucose to rise. Remember, people with type 1 don't make any insulin, and people with type 2 have cells with an attitude!

TYPE 2 DIABETES AND ADOLESCENCE

Unfortunately, there has recently been an increase in the diagnosis of type 2 diabetes in overweight teenagers. That's probably because we as a society have become less active and, as a result, are more overweight. Being overweight, as you recall, contributes to those body cells developing an attitude! For some reason (most likely genetics) there also seems to be more type 2 diabetes diagnosed in African American, Native American, and Hispanic young people as well.

Diabetes really doesn't care who you are, what you do for a living, who your parents are, or where you live. It is a disease that is color-blind, and it will attack both the young and old. Diabetes is found in European countries like Spain, France, and England. It's also found in the Scandinavian countries of Finland and Sweden, in the forests of Africa, or in the northern regions of Alaska and Canada. So you see, wherever you go, chances are there will be people with diabetes.

However, as mentioned previously, there are certain ethnic populations that are at higher risk for developing diabetes. That's because some populations have certain traits (genes) or risk factors that are associated with the development of diabetes. For example, Native Americans, African Americans, Hispanic Americans, Asians, and South Pacific Islanders are all populations that tend to develop type 2 diabetes at disproportionate rates to the general population. You might be thinking, "Why is that?" Well, again those family genes certainly play a major role. But, there are other things that set the stage for the development of diabetes as well. For example, certain customs or lifestyles can increase a person's risk for developing diabetes. What that means is if, for example, you are an African American who has one or both parents with diabetes, maybe a grandmother or an aunt with the disease as well, you know the genes are there! And let's say, as part of your family *custom* you enjoy a home-cooked meal every Sunday with the rest of the family. The meal that you enjoy is based on traditional family recipes with a lot of high fat foods. Unfortunately, this scenario increases the risk for all your family members to develop type 2 diabetes because of the potential for gaining extra weight. You see, the environment that a person lives in also plays a big role in the development of diabetes.

WHAT CAN YOU DO TO DECREASE YOUR FAMILY'S RISK?

So, how can you decrease your family's risk for developing diabetes? There is a lot you can do! First, see a dietitian who can help you and your family members convert your traditional ethnic meals, which may be high in saturated fat, into healthy meals. That's not to say that all ethnic meals are unhealthy or that you need to stop having those family meals! That couldn't be further from the truth. But, for those dishes that are high in fat, there are ways to substitute ingredients to make them a better choice, without sacrificing taste!

Next, if your family isn't already enjoying physical activity, get them moving! For example, there are many wonderful cultural dances and creative physical activities that you and your family members could participate in on a regular basis. That way they will improve their quality of life all on their own! Or if your family has a strong spiritual belief system, go to the elders at your place of worship and tell them that you need help promoting a healthy lifestyle for your family and your community! That will really get your family's attention!

Sometimes though, there are cultural beliefs that discourage or even prevent people from improving their health. For example, within certain Native American populations it may be considered taboo for one to put his or her health needs first over the needs of the family.[12] This is where you really have to turn to the traditions and respected leaders of your culture to seek guidance.

However, keep in mind, there are ways to maintain cultural traditions and still gain health benefits. It just takes someone with strength and innovative ideas! For example, some cultures believe that no matter what they do or don't do, they will surely die from diabetes, because other family members have already died from the disease. This is referred to as fatalism.[13] However, remember attitude can change the world! And attitude can change the outcome of a disease process! The key here is to get your family and your community to talk about it. Get help from your cultural leaders. Encourage them to talk with healthcare professionals to learn ways to improve the health of the people without giving up basic cultural beliefs and traditions. This is a big thing! But, it's worth the effort.

NOTES

1. Joan MacCracken and Donna Hoel, "Puzzles and Promises in Diabetes Management," *Post Graduate Medicine* 101, no. 4 (April 1997), available at www.postgradmed.com/issues/1997/04_97/diabetes.htm (December 27, 2001).

2. Robert Dinsmoor, "Strange Stories," *C.F.K. Magazine* 1996, available at www.jdf.org/kids/searchforacure/2000/0.html (December 27, 2001).

3. MacCracken and Hoel, "Puzzles and Promises in Diabetes Management."

4. Dinsmoor, "Strange Stories."

5. MacCracken and Hoel, "Puzzles and Promises in Diabetes Management."

6. Dinsmoor, "Strange Stories."

7. Luther B. Travis, *An Instructional Aid on Insulin-dependent Diabetes Mellitus* (Austin, Tex.: Designer's Ink, 1999), 25.

8. Peter H. Chase, "What Is Diabetes?" *Understanding Insulin Dependent Diabetes* (2000), available at www.uchsc.edu/misc/diabetes/chap2.html (December 27, 2001).

9. Chase, "What Is Diabetes?"

10. Chase, "What Is Diabetes?"

11. National Institute of Health (March 13, 2002), "Studies to Address Obesity-Linked Diabetes in Children," available at http://www.nichd.nih.gov/new/releases/obese.cfm (November 26, 2002).

12. Mary Annette Pember, "Diabetes among American Indians," *Winds of Change* 17 (Summer 2002): 21.

13. Pember, "Diabetes among American Indians," 22.

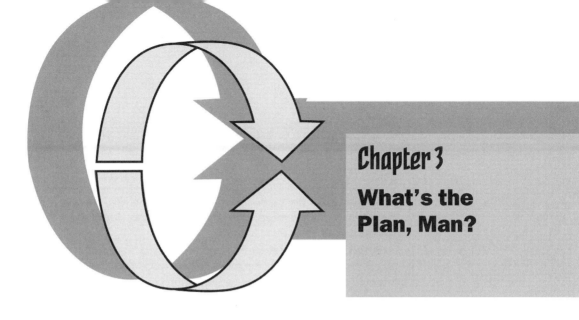

Chapter 3
What's the Plan, Man?

Okay, now what? You've been told you have diabetes, what can you do about it? Well, the good news is there is a lot *you* can do about it! But, first things first, let's talk about what you need to know. You should find out as much as you can about how *you* can manage this yourself. Yeah, you! That doesn't mean you should study to become an endocrinologist (a diabetes specialist) or anything. It just means that you need to hook up with someone in the medical profession whom you trust to give you accurate information about diabetes and how to manage it properly.

A good place to start is with your physician. There are a lot of programs or classes out there that are designed specifically for people with diabetes. And don't worry; these classes aren't like school or anything. The health care *gurus* call them *classes* because they can't come up with anything better to call them! Anyway, they will give you all the basic information that you'll need to know to make your life easier and to keep you healthy! Think of this diabetes plan as a giant puzzle. The diabetes classes just help you make sure all the pieces fit together right! You're probably thinking: "I don't need anyone telling me how to live my life. . . . I have it under control. . . . I've got it all together."

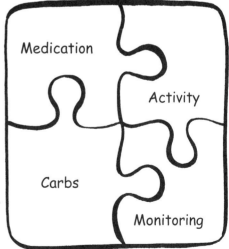

Great! Just for giggles, go to one of these places to see if there is anything out there that would make your life easier. Can't lose; nothing invested but a little time.

EVER WONDER WHERE INSULIN CAME FROM?

Well, soon after the connection between the pancreas and diabetes was discovered, scientists started treating diabetes with pancreatic "extracts."

George Ludwig Zuelzer was one of the first "extractors." He was a young internist in Berlin. In the early 1900s, Zuelzer injected a compound he called "acomatrol" into a dying diabetic patient. The patient improved but later died when Zuelzer's acomatrol supply ran out.[1]

In 1911, a European pharmaceutical company funded Zuelzer, but results were poor. Eventually Zuelzer's lab was turned over to the military during World War I.

At around the same time, Dr. John James Rickard Macleod at the University of Toronto hired Frederick Banting (who asked Charles Herbert Best to assist him) to experiment with pancreatic extracts in dogs. Banting and Best eventually discovered what is now known as insulin.[2]

SO, EXACTLY WHAT DOES THIS PUZZLE INVOLVE?

If you're wondering what this puzzle involves, we can take a little time to go over some of the pieces and look at how they fit together. Let's start with medication. Remember earlier we

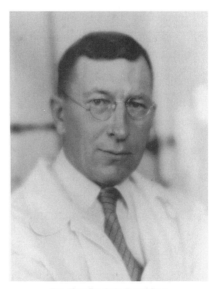

Dr. Frederick Banting

talked about the pancreas and how it is supposed to make insulin? Well, part of the management of type 1 diabetes, and sometimes in type 2 diabetes, includes learning about oral medications and exogenous insulin (which simply means insulin that is provided from outside the body), how it works, and how to get it into your body so it can do what it is supposed to do. Basically, we're just talking about substituting artificial insulin for the insulin that your body *would* make normally if it could (type 1 diabetes) or giving you medication to help your body better use the insulin it already makes or help your body make more of its own insulin (type 2 diabetes). Right now the only way we can give insulin is in the form of a shot, but eventually there will be different ways available to give insulin. We'll talk more about that later.

Insulin in the form of an injection (shot) works a couple of different ways, depending on the type of insulin. So, that means part of the puzzle involves finding the *recipe* of insulin that works best to keep your blood glucose levels within *your* identified target range, regardless of the type of diabetes you have. Yes, that means you and your healthcare provider decide where to set the target. Remember, the target range is important because it not only helps you feel good now, it also helps to make sure you feel good later—way later—like when you're really old! Cool, huh? Just another reason why it's important to find someone you trust who will be able to help you figure out what target range will work best for you.

Now, as far as getting insulin into your body is concerned, that's also something you have control over. You already know you will have to take insulin in the form of

Medication

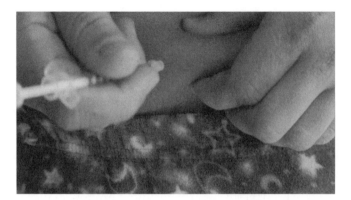

a shot, but there are a lot of different delivery devices you can pick from to do that. For example, there are insulin pens, insulin injectors (no needle, just uses air to push the insulin through your skin!), traditional needle and syringe, and even insulin pumps. There are also regular-size insulin needles, short insulin needles, and really skinny insulin needles. So you see, the choice is yours. Sound confusing? Don't worry, remember there are a lot of people out there who have experience with this stuff; they will be there to help you sort it all out. You just have to hookup with one of them!

Now if you have type 2 diabetes and take oral medication, the same is true for you as well. The key will be to find the *recipe* of medication that will work best to keep your blood glucose levels within *your* identified target range. We'll spend more time talking about all of the different types of medication that are sometimes used to help adolescents with type 2 diabetes a little later.

WHAT CAN I EAT?

Now let's talk about that all important meal plan. Today most people count carbohydrates as a method of maintaining their meal plan. They count carbohydrates (sometimes referred to simply as *carbs*) because it's the carbohydrates in foods that have the biggest effect on blood glucose levels. Sounds weird, but it's really just a simple way to figure out how much food you need to eat to stay healthy and keep your blood glucose levels at target range. No pressure, relax—really you can do this!!! The whole idea is to try to match the amount of glucose in your blood with the amount of insulin you take or with the insulin your body is already making. That way your body will always use the food you are eating for energy and necessary body functions. Dietitians have the most experience with carb counting. So, ask your physician or healthcare professional for the name of a dietitian you can talk to about your meal plan.

Carbs

When you go to see the dietitian, make sure you are honest with him or her. That means making sure you don't hold back anything. This is your opportunity to get what *you* want from this meeting. Remember, this is all about *you*! Some people go in to see the dietitian and say exactly what they think the dietitian wants to hear. Like, "Oh, I love spinach and whole grains; and I never eat anything that isn't nutritious." Yeah right! We're all human! Every once in a while (if not more often!) all of us eat something that isn't nutritious. But the good news is that's okay! As long as most of the time you follow the plan, chances are you will stay healthy. Besides, there is a way to work *all* foods (good and not so good) into your plan. It's all about eating everything in moderation. That means there's no reason to avoid having someone help you figure out what will work for you. Remember, we are all unique individuals and we all have different likes and dislikes. It really does take the help of someone with some experience to figure out all of this stuff. No sense in reinventing the wheel!

In order to develop an individual meal plan, the dietitian will need to have a good idea of the foods you really like to eat and what eating patterns you tend to follow as well. For example, the best thing to do is to go in and tell the dietitian what you prefer. Like, "I really don't eat breakfast, I know I am supposed to, but I just don't like to eat breakfast." Or maybe, "Yeah, I like to eat breakfast, as a matter of fact I really eat a huge breakfast." This can all be worked out in your meal plan. The dietitian will also want to know what kinds of foods you like to eat. So, tell him or her what your favorite foods really are. If you want to work cookies into your meal plan, tell the dietitian that you absolutely love cookies and need to have cookies in your meal plan once in a while. The dietitian will be able to work the cookies into the plan. See, it's not so much the *kinds* of foods you eat, as it is the *amount* of foods you eat. That's because if you eat a lot of food at one time, it can really affect your blood glucose level.

Don't get me wrong, no one is going to say that it's okay to have cookies and cakes and candy every day of the week. That's not healthy—for *anyone*! But, remember the point of the visit with the dietitian is to get a good idea of *your* food preferences and lifestyle. So, don't forget to mention your schedule too. You know things like, if you're the type of person who gets up early, has a busy day all day long, and then goes to bed late. All of these factors need to be thought about when working out the plan, because they will have a big impact on your blood glucose level and the choices you make, for example, deciding what kinds of foods you're going to eat and when you're going to eat them.

Which brings to mind something we talked about earlier—this carb counting thing. The dietitian will talk to you about foods you eat that are primarily made up of carbohydrates, because those are the foods that have the greatest impact on your blood glucose level. Foods like starches, pastas, grains, cereals, fruit, and even sweets are all made up primarily of carbohydrates. Your body uses 100 percent of the carbohydrates in these foods for energy. All of the carbohydrates are turned into glucose and carried through the blood to the cells of the body, where it is used for energy.

Foods that are primarily made up of protein or fat have less effect on blood glucose levels. That's because the body can only use about 40–50 percent of protein for energy. Protein is really supposed to be used to build muscle and repair tissue. Fat is an even more inefficient source of energy. The body can only use about 10 percent of fat for energy. So, now you can see why most of the focus in your meal plan should be on how many carbohydrates (or carbs) are in the foods you choose.

As mentioned previously, part of the dietitian's job is to look at those carbs and to determine how many carb *choices* or how many grams of carbohydrates you should have at each meal (we'll talk about carb choices down the road). The dietitian will also tell you about how much protein and fat is needed for each meal. It's really important to watch the amount of fat in the meal because of the effect fat has on the body. You know, if you eat too much fat, or even eat too much food at one time, it will be stored as fat. And that's not a good thing because it just makes it harder for you to do things—like walk around, breathe, and everything else. And not only that, certain kinds of fat clog up your blood vessels too!

Another thing to keep in mind when you go to see the dietitian is that he or she will not or should not tell you that there are particular foods you *cannot* have. For example, no one should ever tell you that you can't have pizza or ice cream again. If that happens then run!!! Find another dietitian, because that is not the way the meal plan is supposed to work. We now know that we have to be realistic. We know that a meal plan must include all of your favorite foods (maybe not all day, everyday, but in a healthy way, like everyone should eat) in order to ensure that you have a positive experience and are able to follow the plan! So again, when you see the dietitian be honest about the way you eat and the foods you like to eat. Tell that person you definitely love to eat fast food with your friends once a week so he or she can show you how to work that into your meal plan the right way. Great! Right?! Okay!!! After the meal plan is worked out, then you and your healthcare provider will look at your medication needs. You'll go back to that medication puzzle to make sure your insulin matches when your blood glucose is rising after your meals and snacks. Hopefully now you can see how this puzzle starts to come together. Your food and your body's insulin really do

Medication

Carbs

need to *work* together. One more thing about the dietitian, don't think about this whole process as being some kind of a punishment for having diabetes. You know, those thoughts that creep into your head that make you feel that because you have diabetes you'll have to be on a *diet* for the rest of your life! Trust me, no one is going to put you on a *diet*! What we've been talking about is a *meal plan*, not a diet. It is called a meal plan because it is a way of matching, as we said before, your body's insulin levels with your carbohydrate intake. That's why it's important to count carbs; so the insulin and carbohydrates peak in the blood at the same time, allowing the carbohydrates to be used by the body for energy.

Now that we've talked about a couple of pieces of the puzzle, in particular the meal plan and the medication, we know that somehow we have to match what we eat with the proper amount of insulin and/or medication. But, there is another part of the puzzle that also has an effect on blood glucose levels, and that's physical activity. Notice we didn't use the "E" word (exercise)! That's because for some reason when people hear the word *exercise* they freak out! They really get this "I am not going to do this" look on their faces. You've probably seen that look before. Anyway, you can tell by looking at them that the thought of exercise isn't being received well. Think about exercise as just an increase in physical activity. This is really important because when you're active it helps your body use the glucose that's in your blood easier. And because your body can use the glucose easier, you are able to maintain your target glucose level easier.

Activity

So, think about it for a minute. If you do some type of physical activity every day, your body will be able to use the glucose that's in your blood easier, which means you'll get more bang for your buck! This brings to mind an important safety point. If your body is using glucose easier during and after you exercise (oops, increased activity!), then you need to make sure your blood glucose level is in a safe range before you begin any physical activity. You also need to make sure you have some form of carbohydrate available in case your blood glucose drops too low during or immediately after the activity (yes, that can happen). This is primarily a concern for people who take insulin; however, it can also be a concern for people who take oral medication that stimulates your body to make more insulin (more about that later). Keep in mind that the more intense the activity, the more carbohydrates you will need to eat in order to sustain the activity safely. That's where the healthcare professional comes in, because he or she can help you figure out that part of the puzzle. In other words, he or she can help you figure out what it is you need to do so that you can participate in the activity safely.

Maybe you're thinking, "What do you mean *safe*? I don't need any help staying *safe* when I exercise!" Let's clarify that statement. If you're off doing some really strenuous activity all by yourself and your blood glucose level starts to drop, you could have a serious problem. Remember one thing—*prevention* is the key! You've gotta have a plan. You have to know what to do to prevent this from happening. And if by chance it happens anyway (you know—what can happen, will happen!), then you need to have a plan to correct the situation (which includes having carbohydrates available to treat the low blood glucose). We talk more about what to do to prevent and treat low blood glucose in chapter 4.

That brings us to the last piece of the puzzle in diabetes self-management, which is blood glucose monitoring. This piece of the puzzle is a very important piece as well. Did you know that years ago blood glucose monitors weren't available for people to use at home? It's true. People with diabetes used to have to check their urine to see if there was any glucose present, which really only showed if the blood glucose level was high *sometime* before the urine test. The urine test was done by dipping a stick with a special type of a reagent pad on the end of it into a cup

Monitoring

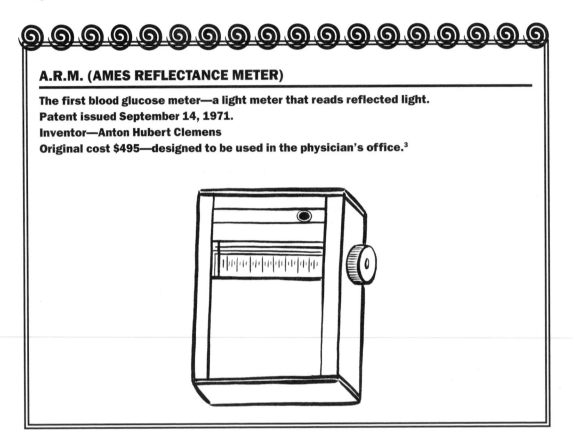

A.R.M. (AMES REFLECTANCE METER)

The first blood glucose meter—a light meter that reads reflected light.
Patent issued September 14, 1971.
Inventor—Anton Hubert Clemens
Original cost $495—designed to be used in the physician's office.[3]

of urine. The pad would then change colors based on the amount of glucose in the urine. The more glucose in the urine, the darker the color would get. The person with diabetes would then compare the color of the pad to a color chart. He or she would then try to "estimate" what the blood glucose *was*. That's because extra glucose in the body is excreted through the urine (you already knew that, right?). When the kidneys recognize that there's too much glucose in the blood during the filtration process, they dump the extra glucose in the urine to try to get rid of it. The only problem with this method of determining the blood glucose level is that it shows what the blood glucose level *was* several hours before (because it takes time for the kidneys to make urine), not what the blood glucose level is *now*. And it's only an estimate. This method of glucose monitoring was certainly nowhere near as accurate as the blood glucose monitors we use today!

Speaking of blood glucose monitors, around 1980 or so, blood glucose monitors became available to the general public. These machines were able to check a person's blood sample to determine the amount of glucose present at any given point in time. This was truly a great improvement that really helped people with diabetes manage their disease more effectively. But you should have seen these monitors when they first came out! They were these huge, monstrous machines! To make it worse, the early monitors required a "hanging drop" of blood. So in order to get enough blood samples for the machine to work properly, people had to literally lance their fingers. It really wasn't all that bad actually, but it just seems very archaic compared to what we have now! It was certainly a big advancement in management, but they were huge (comparatively speaking), and they were really only used in the hospital setting or physician office initially.

Fortunately, with technology and time, researchers finally developed and streamlined these machines so that they became much smaller, faster, and more convenient. And the more advanced they became, the less blood they required!! Most machines on the market today require just a tiny drop of

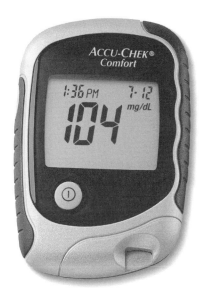

Accu-Chek Advantage Meter courtesy of Roche Diagnostics

blood, which is wonderful compared to the hanging drop of blood that was needed when these machines first came out.

So having this technology available in this day and age is really a benefit. Because of the monitors that we now have available for home use, we can go in, grab a sample of blood, and see what the blood glucose level is right now. That's important, because if you know what the blood glucose is now, you can identify blood glucose patterns and make necessary changes in your treatment plan. In other words, you can look at several days or several readings and discover problems that need your attention. For example, maybe every day at lunchtime you notice that your blood glucose is low. You then need to become a *detective* and try to figure out what might be causing your blood glucose level to drop too low before lunch. If you're maintaining a consistent meal plan, taking your medication consistently in the correct amounts, and have not changed your physical activity, then you know there is something in your plan that needs to be changed. Or conversely, if you notice that your blood glucose is only elevated before a specific meal (just remember, never change your plan based on one blood glucose reading—you need to identify a pattern!) and you know you are consistent with your plan and you haven't changed anything (like the amount of food you're eating or the amount of activity you normally have), then you need to make a change in your current plan. For example, maybe you need to change the amount of carbohydrates you're eating at the meal or snack prior to the elevated reading, or maybe a change in the insulin dose is needed. Once again, this is where that healthcare professional who has some experience identifying blood glucose patterns really can be helpful!

Think of monitoring as a tool. A tool to help you discover how to make these puzzle pieces fit together properly so you stay healthy and feel good. Even though it seems like checking your blood glucose every few hours is a pain (yes, it is), remember the information it gives you is really worth all the trouble. You'll probably agree once you're able to identify your blood glucose patterns and are able to make changes in your management plan. Believe it or not, management really does give you more control over your own life. It just takes time to get used to the idea for one thing, and time to recognize that it really is a small price to pay for the big payoff in the end—and what is the payoff? Well, the payoff for you will be huge in terms of good health right now and even later—twenty, thirty, or even forty years from now. That probably seems like a long time away and you may not be concerned with what happens down the road, but believe it or not, in a blink of an eye you'll be there!

Know your A1c

Another blood test that is important for you to know about is the A1c test. Think of this test as a way of determining your batting average versus how you're doing in the baseball game today. When we talk about blood glucose monitoring, we're not just talking about looking at what your blood glucose is on your home blood glucose monitor (how you're doing in the game today), but also looking at what your average is over a period of several months by looking at your A1c test (your overall batting average!). The A1c test is really important because it tells the big picture.

The A1c test is a cool thing actually. Researchers figured out that they could get a pretty good idea of what a person's *average* blood glucose is by looking at how much glucose is stuck to the red blood cells. See, a red blood cell lives about 120 days or so, then a new red blood cell takes its place. But, what is unique about red blood cells is that they carry hemoglobin, which is how we get oxygen in all the cells of our body. Well, it wasn't long before scientists

Table 3.1.   A1c, what does it mean?

A1c		Glucose (mg/dL)
14.0		360
13.5	**STOP!**	
13.0	**GET HELP**	330
12.5	This is very	
12.0	**SERIOUS!**	300
11.5		
11.0		270
10.5		
10.0		240
9.5	**WARNING!**	
9.0	This is too	210
8.5	**HIGH!**	
8.0	**Getting**	180
7.5	**Better!**	
7.0	(Still a little high)	150
6.5		
6.0	**Just Right!**	120
5.5	(where people without	
5.0	diabetes usually are)	90
4.0		60

figured out that glucose likes to stick to a certain part of the hemoglobin molecule (called the A1c) on the red blood cell. So, by counting the amount of glucose that's stuck to the hemoglobin molecule, scientists are able to determine a person's average blood glucose over the past 120 days (because that's how long the average red blood cell lives). With further research they also found that if a person with diabetes has an average A1c level of 7 percent or less, he or she has much less risk of developing complications of diabetes. What a great discovery! This test has certainly helped people manage their diabetes better over time.

Anyway, getting back to this monitoring piece of the puzzle, you can see why it makes a big difference in your management to have numbers that tell you if what you're doing is working or not. If what you are doing isn't working, then monitoring can also help you identify where you need to fine-tune your management to get back to your target blood glucose goals. Certainly, in order for your life to be easier, all the pieces of the puzzle need to fit together correctly. And that is the whole name of the game. Again that's just another reason why it's important for you to have a healthcare professional who understands how to manage diabetes and who can talk to you in a way that you understand. Even more important, though, make sure you have a healthcare professional that understands you! That way you can work together to make the changes needed to hit those targets! Remember, too, you are really just like everyone else out there; the only difference is you just happen to have diabetes. The whole key to this management thing is to figure out what it is you can do to make your life what you want it to be!

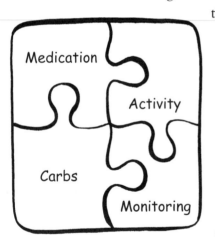

NOTES

1. Joan MacCracken and Donna Hoel, "Puzzles and Promises in Diabetes Management," *Post Graduate Medicine* 101, no. 4 (April

1997), available at www.postgradmed.com/issues/1997/ 04_97/diabetes.htm (December 27, 2001).

2. MacCracken and Hoel, "Puzzles and Promises in Diabetes Management."

3. Rick Mendosa, available at www.Mendosa.com/ (November 21, 2002).

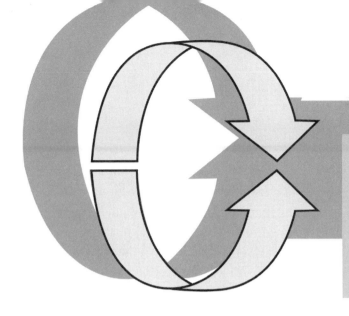

It probably wouldn't be hard to think of about a hundred reasons why you don't want to monitor your blood glucose. Maybe your fingers hurt; it's a pain to carry the equipment around with you all the time; or nobody else has to do it, so why should I? How about the big one—it isn't fair! Well, you know what? It's not fair. But, there is one huge reason why you should monitor. Monitoring your blood glucose will allow you to be *you*! Without a blood glucose monitor, you won't be able to tell if your blood glucose is high or low until you are already having some pretty nasty symptoms. That means you could be driving a car with a low blood glucose level and not even realize it—until it's too late! Now that could really affect your life! Or, your blood glucose level could be high, making you feel really thirsty and causing you to run to the bathroom all the time. How fun would that be? Talk about interfering with your life! Can you imagine being constantly interrupted to go tend to the *call of nature*? Now, if you have a blood glucose monitor (and use it!), you could identify blood glucose patterns, make changes in your management, and decrease the symptoms of the acute complications of diabetes. Yeah!

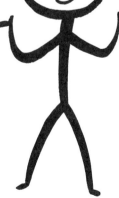

Why should I check my blood glucose?

WHAT ARE THE ACUTE COMPLICATIONS OF DIABETES?

The acute complications of diabetes are high (hyperglycemia) and low (hypoglycemia) blood glucose levels, which really can make

Is monitoring worth it?

you feel crappy. It's no picnic feeling shaky, dizzy, irritable, and not being able to put one foot in front of the other without using extreme brainpower. That's what it feels like to have low blood glucose. Sometimes, if the blood glucose level drops really low, and you can't eat or drink anything to bring it back up on your own (like if you're unconscious), then you'll have to depend on someone else to give you an injection of something called glucagon. Glucagon is a hormone made by the pancreas that stimulates the body to release stored glucose from the liver. This causes the blood glucose level to rise. Keep in mind severe hypoglycemia (low blood glucose) doesn't happen very often. Usually there's a reason for it. Like maybe you wait too long to eat after taking your insulin. This is one acute complication you will want to avoid.

It's also no fun dealing with hyperglycemia (high blood glucose). Think about it, running to the bathroom every hour on the hour when you're at a party or in class can really be a pain! But that's not all; high blood glucose can even mess with your vision. When your blood glucose level is high, sometimes your vision can get blurry or cloudy. It can be different for different people, but regardless, having your vision screwed up, even for a short period of time, can really interfere with your plans! So see, having high and low blood glucose is a pain for a couple of reasons: First you feel like crap; second, you have to deal with the symptoms and the havoc these symptoms cause in your life.

When my blood glucose is low I feel weak and sometimes my mouth feels numb.—Steve

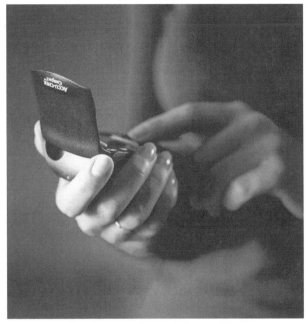

Compact meter courtesy of Roche Diagnostics

I have no energy when my blood glucose is high—and I feel sick to my stomach.—Nikki

SO, WHAT CAN YOU DO?

The good news is that monitoring really gives you some control over all of that. It allows you to figure out what needs to be done to prevent the highs and lows from happening in the first place—and that's the key. So yeah, monitoring is a pain because you have to carry around all that equipment, and yeah you've gotta poke your finger and get a drop of blood, but at least it allows you to live your life the way you want to

33

Monitoring your blood glucose will allow you to be *You*!

live it. And besides, we live in the age of technology! So now there are a lot of different cool monitors out there that even fit different personalities; everything from the traditional monitors to the alternative site monitors. With alternative site monitors you don't even have to prick your finger! You can use your forearm or even the palm of your hand to give your fingers a break. There's also a new monitor that resembles a watch. It checks your blood glucose through a sensor that tests fluid through your skin. One thing to remember about this watch-like monitor is that it has to be calibrated against a blood glucose value obtained from a traditional monitor every twelve hours when the sensor is changed. But, at least it gives you another alternative (which is a good thing)!

How often you check your blood glucose is up to you. But you will get a better idea of what is really going on if you check your blood glucose before each meal and at bedtime. Sometimes it helps if you also check your blood glucose two hours after a meal now and then to see if your blood glucose really is coming back down to your target level after you eat. And of course, there will be times when you'll have to check your blood glucose more frequently. For example, it's a good idea to check more frequently when your body is stressed (illness or injury), when you feel like your blood glucose is low, if your blood glucose has been erratic lately, if you become pregnant, or if you are making changes in your treatment plan.

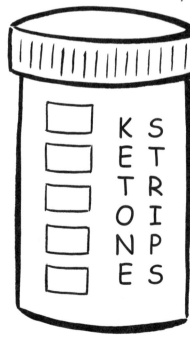

Urine ketone or blood ketone testing is another type of monitoring or testing of which you should be aware. That's primarily done whenever your blood glucose is over 250 mg/dl or 300 mg/dl, like when you're sick with the flu or something. This test checks for the presence of ketone bodies in your urine or blood. Remember earlier we talked about how when your blood glucose level is high, and your body can't use the glucose for energy because there's not enough working insulin, the body looks for an alternative source of energy? And we said that typically the body will try to break down fat for energy first. Now remember, the problem with that is that fat is really an inefficient source of energy. Your body has to break down a lot of fat quickly in order to get enough fuel to meet your body's needs. So, what happens is the body continues to break down fat really fast. And as the body is doing this, the byproduct of the fat breakdown, ketone bodies, starts to build up in the blood. Now, if the body can get rid of the ketones in the blood there is no problem. Unfortunately, because the body is breaking down the fat so fast, sometimes the body can't get rid of the ketones through the urine fast enough. What happens then is ketones start to build up in the blood, which eventually makes the person very sick. This is because ketones are really acids. So when you have an illness, like a cold, and your blood glucose is high, your body is not using the glucose in your blood effectively. That means the likelihood of your body starting to break down fat is present, and you need to check if ketones are present in the urine or blood.

You can do this test very easily by using urine ketone strips. First you'll need to get a urine specimen (no problem when your blood sugar is high!), then you just stick the end of the ketone strip right into the urine sample. There is a little pad on the end of the strip that turns colors when it is exposed to ketones in the urine. All you have to do then is match the color of the strip to the color chart on the side of the bottle to determine your ketone level. The darker the color, the more ketones there are in your urine.

KETONE STRIPS

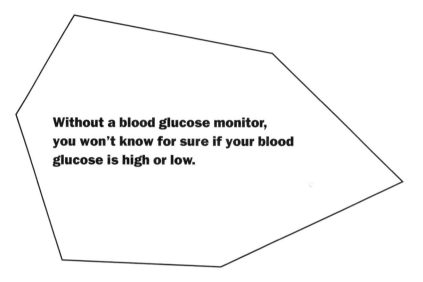

Without a blood glucose monitor, you won't know for sure if your blood glucose is high or low.

That sounds like a really nasty job, doesn't it? But, remember one thing, this little test can keep you out of the hospital. Once you have ketones present in your urine, in moderate to large amounts, you definitely need help from a healthcare professional. The body can usually clear out small amounts of ketones from the blood and prevent acidosis (a condition caused from the extra acid in the blood). But, once your blood has a moderate, or certainly a large amount of ketones, you may start to develop symptoms of ketoacidosis. For example, you may have a stomachache, feel like you want to puke, or there may even be a fruity smell to your urine or breath. Once ketoacidosis develops we know there is a real problem. At that point usually the only thing that is going to help is hospitalization. You will need intravenous fluids (through a vein) and insulin in order to correct the acidic environment that has developed in your body. So again, the key is prevention!

But, if checking for ketones in the urine grosses you out, you can always check for ketones in the blood. That's another alternative that is now available. There are monitors out there that check for both blood glucose and blood ketones through special strips for each. You just put a drop of blood on the strip indicated for blood ketone testing, and then the monitor will calculate the amount of ketones present in the blood. So you can see there is a real purpose for performing all of these tasks in diabetes management; these tools help you keep yourself feeling well and keep you out of the hospital!

WHAT DO I DO WITH THE RESULTS FROM THESE TESTS?

Let's talk about what to do with the results of all these tests. If you are the kind of person who is going to go through all of the trouble of checking your blood glucose level four, five, six times or more a day and then do absolutely nothing with the results, then you're really wasting your time. And you're not doing yourself any good! You really need to learn what to do with these numbers. It's great that you write down all your results everyday (look at table 4.1) or keep the results on your glucose monitor memory, but you need to go one step further and *do something* with the results! What should you do? Well, let's start with a couple of rules of thumb. First, you should never make any changes in your management plan based on only one blood glucose reading. You know that your blood glucose level can literally change from minute to minute throughout any given day. There are many different things that can affect your blood glucose. For example, what you eat certainly affects your blood glucose, but so can stress and hormones that are released in your body throughout the day. So instead of trying to figure things out based on one blood glucose result, you need to look for a pattern. If you notice a pattern that seems to occur around the same time each day, then you know you

Table 4.1. Blood Glucose Log

	M	T	W	Th	F	Sat	Sun
Bkf	120	145	116	182	232	222	145
Lch	98	132	149	122	139	119	108
Dnr	148	154	147	132	145	168	138
Bed	121	114	130	146	133	155	126

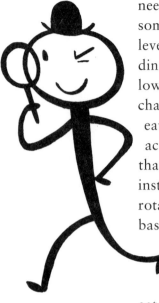

need to do some detective work. Look to see if there is something you are doing that caused your blood glucose level to change. Let's say that for the past two days before dinner you noticed that your blood glucose has been too low. The first thing you need to ask yourself is, "What has changed in my daily routine or daily management?" Are you eating less carbs at lunch or snack? Did you change your activity level? Did you take more insulin or oral medication than usual? Are you rotating insulin injection sites as instructed (insulin can build up in one area if you don't rotate sites, not to mention that insulin absorption varies based on where you give the injection)? If all of these things are unchanged, then you can assume that what you need to change is your management plan. Maybe you need to change your carb amount or the time that you eat. Or maybe you'll need to reevaluate the amount or time you take your insulin.

DO I HAVE TO DO THIS ALONE?

Don't think that you have to do this on your own. Once you learn the principles of diabetes management, you certainly can manage your diabetes if you choose to, because you really will be the expert in *your* diabetes. Remember 95 percent of the care a person receives for diabetes comes from the person with diabetes! Of course, you'll need to see your healthcare professional every three months or so to review your plan and to get help in fine-tuning your management. Just remember, you don't have to be in the management boat alone. There are a lot of healthcare professionals with experience in diabetes management who can help you figure out the puzzle. These professionals are available every day to help you determine the most likely reason your blood glucose is varying, and then help you make the changes needed to get your blood glucose levels back to target.

So you see, you really do have a choice in this. It always comes back to choice, your choice. Can you see the central theme here? Diabetes is the type of disease where *you* can really make a difference in how it affects *your* life. That's because you have control over your management.

If you decide you want to take the road of *progress* and that you want to be the one calling the shots in your diabetes management, then you need to become educated about your disease. Also, keep in mind that you need to use the numbers from your daily monitoring to help you identify patterns (because again you should never change your plan based on one blood glucose reading). And second, remember to do your detective work and try to come up with the most likely reason for the change in your blood glucose levels. Then you will be able to make the adjustments necessary in your management plan to bring your blood glucose levels back down to your desired target goal.

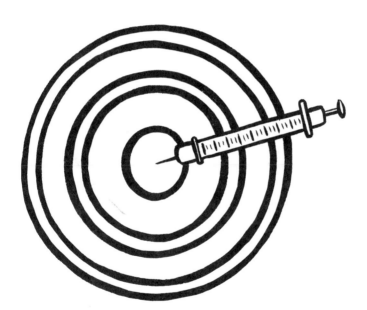

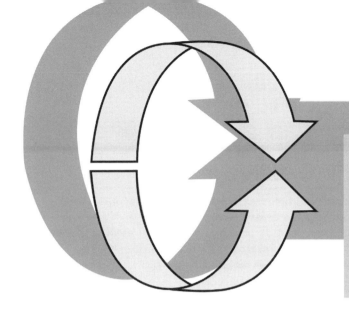

Chapter 5

To Eat and What Not to Eat? That Is the Question!

Okay, by now you probably got the idea that what you eat may really affect your blood glucose level. So let's talk about how that happens, and what you can do to stay ahead of the game. Keep one thing in mind: The goal of meal planning is to help you make decisions that will maintain or improve your diabetes management and help keep you healthy.

So, do you need to follow a meal plan? The answer is a resounding *yes*! It's true, really! Following a plan will help you stay on track and make your life a whole lot easier in the long run. In order to get with the program though, you'll need to see a dietitian who knows about diabetes management. That way, he or she will be able to help you with a plan that fits your lifestyle and one that will help you meet your goals. But remember, this is not a once in a lifetime thing! You will need to review your plan with a dietitian every so often to make adjustments and modify your plan as your life changes. It's also a good idea to have your family members or friends take part in your plan as well. That way you'll have someone for support. Who knows, they may even get some useful information for themselves! But, again that's totally up to you.

Remember what we said before: You don't have to worry that the dietitian is going to try to change your life. You know, like trying to make you eat at times that aren't convenient for you or eat foods that you don't like. The goal in diabetes management is to balance food with medication and activity in order to meet blood glucose targets and maintain health, but it is important to

> ## WHAT'S A CARBOHYDRATE?
>
> - Carbohydrates are a major source of energy for the body.
> - Carbohydrates provide 4 kcal per gram.
> - Approximately 60–70 percent of total daily calories should come from carbohydrates and monosaturated fat.
> - Carbohydrate sources include: sugars (fruit, milk) and starches (bread, cereal).
>
> Sugars do not have more of an effect on blood glucose than starches—the amount of carbohydrates and the amount of food eaten have more effect on blood glucose levels—but, remember foods with more sugar add calories and maybe even fat.

do this by fitting diabetes management into your *usual* routine. No one is going to try to change your life to fit your diabetes management. It makes more sense to fit your diabetes management into your life, doesn't it? However, unless you are using insulin pump therapy or multiple daily injections, you will need to eat similar amounts of food at consistent times that are coordinated with your insulin and/or oral medication action times. Spreading food intake throughout the day with five or six small meals and snacks may be helpful as well.

WHAT WILL THE DIETITIAN DO?

So what can you expect when you see the dietitian? Well, to begin with, the dietitian will gather information that will help both of you determine the best meal plan for your lifestyle. The first meeting usually consists of an assessment in which the dietitian will look at your blood work results (either you can bring these with you or your doctor can send them to the dietitian). He or she will look at things like your cholesterol, fasting blood glucose, A1c, triglycerides (three fatty acids attached to a glycerol molecule), and the results of your urine test for microalbumin (tiny amounts of protein in the urine). In addition, your medical history, blood pressure, and medications will be looked at. The dietitian will also take into account your learning style, culture, religion, and your food-related beliefs and concerns. In order to do this, though, the dietitian will probably ask you to fill out a food and nutrition history. Either you can tell the dietitian what you usually eat when you go for your appointment, or you might be asked to keep a food record for a few days before the appointment. Keep in mind, it's really important for you to keep good records so that you can get the most from your appointment. After the assessment, the dietitian will talk to you about basic nutrition and perhaps about beginning strategies for altering eating patterns if needed (like making good food choices). After you have that down, the dietitian will ask to see you again to give you more in-depth information that includes diabetes management skills. This information is totally individualized based on your preferences, lifestyle, and what you already know. It's during this time that you

IS PROTEIN IMPORTANT? YES!

- Protein is needed for growth, tissue repair, and is a secondary source of energy.
- Protein contributes 4 kcal per gram.
- Approximately 15–20 percent of total daily calories should come from protein sources.
- Sources of protein include: meat, dairy products, legumes, nuts, seeds, and vegetables.

STOP! DON'T EAT TOO MUCH FAT!

- Only a small amount of fat from food is used for energy.
- It's broken down into triglycerides and stored as body fat.
- Fat contributes 9 kcal per gram.
- As mentioned previously, carbohydrates and monosaturated fat (like canola, olive, and peanut oil) should provide 60–70 percent of energy intake.
- Seven to 10 percent of calories or less should come from saturated fat (any fat source that is solid at room temperature—meat, butter, and bacon).
- Ten percent of calories should come from polyunsaturated fat (corn, safflower, soybean, and sunflower oil).
- A diet should include 200–300 mg of cholesterol (found in animal foods) per day or less.
- Trans fatty acids should be avoided.
- Other fat sources include: egg yolk, dairy, margarine, and snack foods (of course!)

will be taught how to make changes in your meal plan for different situations that arise in your life. Remember, flexibility is the key here! So, for example, you'll need to learn how to read food labels, what to do when you're sick, and how to compensate for changes in mealtimes, exercise, or even holidays.

HOW DOES THE DIETITIAN KNOW WHAT I NEED?

So, how does the dietitian determine what and how much you need to eat to stay healthy? Well, that's a good question! Let's look at that. First the dietitian will need to determine your caloric needs. That just means he or she will figure out the amount of calories you will need to maintain a *reasonable* body weight (which depends on several factors, like your level of activity and age). The best way to determine caloric needs, again, is by keeping a complete record of the foods you usually eat. Then he or she will validate your caloric needs based on a formula.

Sometimes, though, the focus of the plan may just be on the amount of carbohydrates needed to maintain glucose control and promote health. This type of meal planning is referred to as carbohydrate counting or simply, carb counting. This is really just about eating a consistent amount of carbohydrate-type foods at consistent times so that the glucose reaches the blood about the same time the insulin is peaking in the blood. Ahh! Now it all makes sense! It really is like a puzzle—and the pieces do need to work together in the right way for it to come out right! This type of meal planning has been around for a long time, since insulin was discovered! So, a lot of people have used this method successfully over the years. It was even used in a research trial called the Diabetes Control

---

CAN YOU BELIEVE THE FAT IN THIS FOOD?

ʃ = 1 teaspoon of fat
Cheeseburger ʃ ʃ ʃ ʃ
French fries (med) ʃ ʃ ʃ ʃ
Fried fish sandwich ʃ ʃ ʃ ʃ ʃ ʃ ʃ
Fried chicken sandwich ʃ ʃ ʃ ʃ ʃ
Onion rings (med) ʃ ʃ ʃ
Wing dings (6) ʃ ʃ ʃ ʃ ʃ ʃ
Fried chicken (white meat) ʃ ʃ ʃ ʃ ʃ
Fried chicken (dark meat) ʃ ʃ ʃ
Chicken nuggets (6) ʃ ʃ ʃ
Pepperoni pizza (1 slice) ʃ ʃ
Beef taco ʃ ʃ
Bean burrito ʃ ʃ
Taco salad with shell ʃ ʃ ʃ ʃ ʃ ʃ ʃ ʃ ʃ ʃ

IT'S ALL IN THE PORTION SIZE . . .

Handful = one cup
Baseball = cup of fruit
One dice = 1 tsp of butter or margarine

DIABETES CONTROL AND COMPLICATIONS TRIAL (DCCT)

- 1983–1993
- 1441 people with type 1 diabetes participated.
- Involved 29 clinical centers in the United States and Canada, and eight central laboratories and units participated in the trial.
- Showed that tight control of blood glucose levels can decrease and/or prevent the complications of diabetes.
- Tight control included: Testing blood glucose levels four or more times a day; four daily insulin injections or use of an insulin pump; adjustment of insulin doses according to food intake and exercise; a diet and exercise plan; monthly visits to a healthcare team composed of a physician, nurse educator, dietitian, and behavioral therapist.

and Complications Trial (DCCT) that was instrumental in demonstrating how diabetes self-care management (that's really what we've been talking about all this time) can improve the health of a person with diabetes and even prevent or delay complications. Not only that, but other research studies have shown that it is really the carbohydrates that have an effect on the blood glucose level after a meal anyway. That's why there's been so much attention on carbs

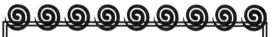

IT'S ALL IN THE PORTION SIZE . . .

Clenched small fist = ½ cup
Thumb = 1 ounce
Thumb tip = 1 tsp
Palm of hand = 3 oz of meat

recently! But, what's really great about carb counting is that it gives you more flexibility, while helping with glucose control! On the flip side though, carb counting does call for more blood glucose monitoring and decision making from you. However, you can't just ignore the amount of fat and protein in the food you eat either. If you do, you could really end up gaining a lot of weight. Given all that, let's talk about what carb counting involves. There are three levels in carb counting. We'll talk about each of these levels individually.

LEVEL ONE

Level one is the beginning or basic level that is concerned mostly about eating consistent amounts of carbohydrates at each meal and snack in order to reduce fluctuations in blood glucose levels. So, the dietitian will help you identify which foods contain carbohydrates, what portion size equals a carbohydrate choice (one serving of carbohydrate), and how to find and use carbohydrate information. For example, you'll learn that one carbohydrate choice is equal to about 15 grams of carbohydrate. Let's see, that would be the same as one small apple or orange, or one cup of milk, or even one slice of bread. See carb counting gives you more choices, and really it's not all that hard either. Remember though, the only way you'll be able to tell if your plan is working will be through blood glucose monitoring.

LEVEL TWO

Level two is where you'll learn the connection between food, medication, activity, and blood glucose (which is also known as pattern management). For this level you'll need a calculator (unless you're good at doing math in your head) to help you do some simple calculations to determine the carbohydrate content of the food you're eating. You'll also learn how to read food labels and determine the role of protein, fat, and fiber in carbohydrate counting. Then you'll learn pattern management as you start to identify patterns related to what you're eating, the amount of insulin you're taking, the amount of activity you're participating in, and how these factors are affecting your blood glucose.

LOOK AT THE AMOUNT OF SUGAR IN THIS FOOD!

ꟾ = 1 teaspoon of sugar
12 oz regular pop ꟾꟾꟾꟾꟾꟾꟾꟾꟾ
20 oz regular pop ꟾꟾꟾꟾꟾꟾꟾꟾꟾꟾꟾꟾ
2-liter regular pop ꟾꟾꟾꟾꟾꟾꟾꟾꟾꟾ
ꟾꟾꟾꟾꟾꟾꟾꟾꟾꟾꟾꟾꟾꟾꟾꟾꟾꟾꟾ
ꟾꟾꟾꟾꟾꟾꟾꟾꟾꟾꟾꟾꟾ

LEVEL THREE

And finally level three is the advanced level of carbohydrate counting that teaches you how to match insulin to carbohydrate intake using a ratio. This is the level that you'll use for multiple daily injections or for insulin pump therapy. The main thing you'll have to do here is accurately estimate the amount of carbohydrates you're eating. That way you'll be able to give yourself rapid or fast acting insulin to cover the carbohydrate load based on your individualized insulin to carb ratio. The insulin to carb ratio is based on how your body responds to a glucose load. In other words, how much insulin it will take to bring your blood glucose to target level after a meal. But keep in mind that the carb to insulin ratio can change with a change in body weight or even physical activity. In addition, you may have a different carb to insulin ratio that you use based on the meal. That's because your body can be more or less sensitive to insulin based on the time of day, due to the influence of hormones that are released during that part of the day. For example, in the morning the carb to insulin ratio may need to be *less* because of the influence of counterregulatory hormones like glucagon, cortisol, growth hormone, epinephrine, and norepinephrine. As a result of these hormones, the body needs more insulin to do the same job, creating the need for a *lower* carb to insulin ratio (which really means you need more insulin to cover the carbohydrate load). Sound confusing? Well, with practice it really does become second nature. And don't worry, there are plenty of people out there who are experts in figuring this stuff out, and they will help you.

Table 5.1.   Macaroni and Cheese Food Label

Macaroni and Cheese
Nutrition Facts

Serving Size 1 cup (228 g)
Servings Per Container 2

Amount Per Serving

Calories 260   Calories from Fat 120

	% Daily Value*
Total fat 13g	20%
Saturated Fat 5g	25%
Cholesterol 30mg	10%
Sodium 660mg	28%
Total Carbohydrate 31g	10%
Dietary Fiber 0g	0%
Sugars 5g	
Protein 5g	

1 cup of macaroni and cheese =
31 g Carbohydrate and 13 g Fat

Remember—Sugar-free and fat free do not mean "carb free."

One more thing, you'll have to be careful not to overeat!
Because of the flexibility that comes with carbohydrate
counting, you could gain weight by eating more than your body
needs. Remember, you're just like everyone else, if you eat too
much you'll gain weight! There will be other issues that the
dietitian will address with you as needed, like how fat affects
stomach-emptying time for example (slows it down, causing a
delay in the blood glucose peak, which needs to be matched to
your body's insulin peak). But, don't freak out! You will get it
with some practice. It just takes time.

WHAT ABOUT ARTIFICIAL SWEETENERS?

Fact: Saccharin, aspartame (Equal®), acesulfame K, and
sucralose (Splenda®) have all been approved by the Food and
Drug Administration (FDA) for use by people with diabetes in
the United States.

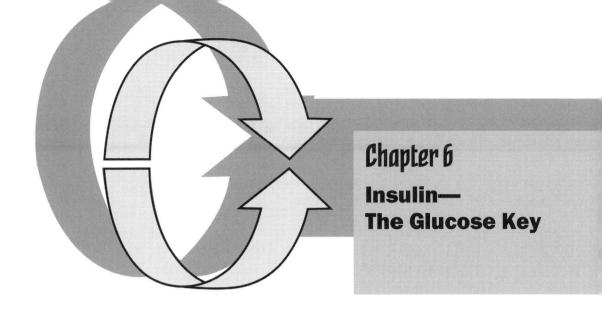

Chapter 6
Insulin—
The Glucose Key

Insulin is a hormone that's made by the pancreas in direct proportion to the amount of glucose in the blood. Remember how insulin pairs up with glucose in the blood and travels together with the glucose to the cell? Well, when the insulin and the glucose get to the cell the insulin changes the cell membrane, allowing the glucose to move into the cell where it can be used for energy. You can also think of insulin as a key. The insulin key opens the door on the cell and allows the glucose to enter, mix with oxygen, and cause those tiny little bursts of energy to occur. So, it's easy to understand why, without insulin, people with diabetes are not able to use the glucose in their blood and end up having symptoms of high blood glucose.

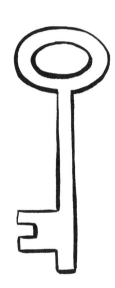

TYPE 1 DIABETES

With type 1 diabetes, the person no longer has any functioning beta cells left in the pancreas to make insulin. You know that everybody has a pancreas; well everybody also has tiny cells in the pancreas called *beta cells* that are located in the *islets of Langerhans* (in the tail of the pancreas). The beta cells actually make the hormone insulin. Remember earlier when we talked about type 1 diabetes? We said that scientists think that type 1 diabetes develops when the body is exposed to an environmental trigger that causes the body to destroy its own beta cells. For example, one theory suggests that the body is exposed to a virus that looks very similar to the beta cells.

When the body makes antibodies in response to the invading virus and starts to fight it off, it mistakes the beta cells as the invading virus, because they look so much alike. So, when the body gets rid of the virus, it gets screwed up and gets rid of the beta cells at the same time. This causes the person to have what is known as a *complete lack* of insulin production (no longer able to make insulin) and he or she develops type 1 diabetes. As a result, there's a rapid increase in the blood glucose level because there is no place for the glucose to go. The symptoms again may include extreme thirst, frequent trips to the bathroom, and feeling very tired and hungry (because without glucose, the cells get tired and hungry).

TYPE 2 DIABETES

Now with type 2 diabetes, the process and the cause for high blood glucose are a little different. Remember, people with type 2 diabetes still have beta cells that are making insulin. The problem is that their bodies are making insulin keys that don't work! See, the body still makes insulin based on the amount of glucose in the blood, pairs it up with the glucose, and both eventually find their way to the cells. But, when the insulin gets to the cell, it's confronted by a cell with an attitude! The cells don't allow the insulin to do its job. It's as if the cells think the insulin is the wrong key. As a result, the person ends up in the same situation as a person without functioning beta cells, even though he or she has beta cells that are working. That's because without insulin that *works* properly, the glucose stays in the blood stream, causing the symptoms of high blood glucose. Remember, when the glucose can't leave the blood and go into the cells where it is needed for energy, it has to stay in the blood stream until it is excreted from the body. That, my friend, is what causes the signs and symptoms of high blood glucose— running to the bathroom all the time, feeling very thirsty, very tired, and ultimately getting dehydrated as the body tries to get rid of the extra glucose in the blood through the urine.

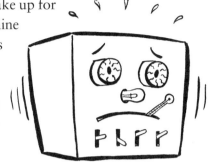

Eventually the body tries to make extra insulin to make up for the insulin that isn't working. But, just like any machine that works too long and too hard, the pancreas starts to get slower and slower until it can't make enough insulin to meet the body's needs. This causes what is known as a *relative lack of insulin*, which just means that there's insulin being made in the body, but there isn't enough insulin to meet the body's needs.

WHAT HAPPENS WHEN INSULIN ISN'T AVAILABLE?

So, what happens when a person isn't making any insulin (type 1 diabetes) or when a person makes insulin, but it just doesn't work right (type 2 diabetes)? Well, with type 1 diabetes the person must take insulin injections for the rest of his or her life in order to live. With type 2 diabetes, usually meal planning, physical activity, and/or oral medications work just fine. But sometimes even with type 2 diabetes these may not be enough to keep the blood glucose at the target level. In this situation, even though the person is making insulin, the treatment includes insulin injections in order to bring the glucose level

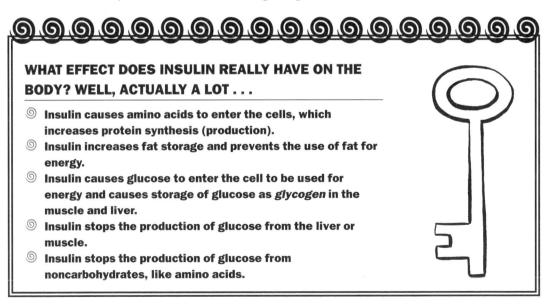

WHAT EFFECT DOES INSULIN REALLY HAVE ON THE BODY? WELL, ACTUALLY A LOT . . .

- Insulin causes amino acids to enter the cells, which increases protein synthesis (production).
- Insulin increases fat storage and prevents the use of fat for energy.
- Insulin causes glucose to enter the cell to be used for energy and causes storage of glucose as *glycogen* in the muscle and liver.
- Insulin stops the production of glucose from the liver or muscle.
- Insulin stops the production of glucose from noncarbohydrates, like amino acids.

down. In other words, people with type 2 diabetes don't take insulin because they are not making insulin; they take it because all the other treatments available don't bring the blood glucose levels down enough to prevent the complications of diabetes. As a result, they need to take insulin in the form of an injection to stay healthy. But, as you can see, with either type of diabetes, insulin can certainly be the *key* to maintaining health and well-being.

Unfortunately, the only way we can currently give insulin is in the form of an injection (a shot). That's because insulin is a protein. So, if a person with diabetes were to swallow an "insulin pill," enzymes in the stomach would break it down similar to the way protein in food is broken down. As a result, the insulin would never be able to do its job because it would never actually get into the bloodstream and into the cells to work.[1] That's why insulin has to be given in the form of an injection, so it can bypass the digestion process and get right to the bloodstream where it can be taken to all of the cells of the body. However, it may interest you to know that researchers are currently working on an insulin pill! They're trying to put a *secret coating* around the insulin so that it can get through the stomach without being detected! But don't get too excited, there's still a lot of work to do before it's ready to test on people.

You may also be wondering, "If I take oral medication to help keep my blood glucose in control, and these pills aren't insulin, then what are they?" Good question! The pills used to control the blood glucose level in people with type 2 diabetes work on different parts of the body to either help the body's insulin work better or help the body make more insulin on its own. You'll have a chance to learn all about these medications in the next chapter.

WHAT DO YOU NEED TO KNOW?

Okay, so what do you need to know about insulin? Well, let's talk about that. First you need to know that there are different types of insulin, different concentrations of insulin, and even different sources of insulin! Primarily there are two sources of insulin available now in the United States. One is a human source and the other is an animal source. The insulin from animal sources is isolated from beef and pork pancreas glands. However, the animal sources are slowly being discontinued because there is more insulin antibody formation noted with animal sources. This antibody formation may alter the predictability of the insulin's peak effect and duration of action (we'll talk about what this is in a minute) and even cause more of a localized reaction than is noted with human insulin.[2]

In case you're wondering, human insulin does not come from a human being. In other words, we don't take insulin from one person and give it to another person. It's called human insulin because it more closely *resembles* true human insulin. Instead, human insulin is made from bacteria (E coli) or fungal cells (Saccharomyces cerevisiae), or by using recombinant-DNA technology (biosynthetic). This type of insulin is an option for vegetarians, Muslims, Orthodox Jews, or Hindus who prefer not to use pork or beef insulin.[4] However, human insulin can also be made through a chemical conversion process using pork insulin (semisynthetic), and that's important to know as well.

THE FIRST INSULIN

- Banting and Best, physiologists working at the University of Toronto, discovered that they could make active insulin in 1921.
- This new insulin was first given to a human being in January 1922 in Canada.
- The insulin that was used in those early years caused a big drop in the number of deaths from diabetic coma and it even increased how long people lived after being diagnosed with diabetes.
- However, this insulin also caused sudden drops in blood glucose (hypoglycemia). So, new forms of insulin were developed that acted slower.
- One such insulin, developed by Hagedorn of Denmark in 1936, used protamine, a protein-like substance, which made it start working slower and last longer.
- We know this insulin today as NPH insulin.[3]

HOW IS INSULIN CLASSIFIED?

Insulin is classified according to peak effect (when it's working the hardest) and duration of action (how long it works). Aren't you glad you asked? See, insulin is really very similar to, for example, the kids in your class or your friends;

INSULIN PREPARATION

1. **Gather your supplies.**
2. **Wash your hands.**
3. **Roll the insulin.**
4. **Pull the syringe plunger down until the top of the plunger is in line with the dose to be taken (need to put air in the bottle before you can draw up your dose).**
5. **With the bottle of insulin sitting on a flat surface, insert the needle and push the air into the bottle.**
6. **Turn the bottle upside down leaving the syringe in the bottle, and pull down on the plunger past the dose you want to draw up (two to four units past is fine).**
7. **Check for air bubbles (these do not hurt you, but they do take up space that is supposed to be used for insulin).**
8. **If bubbles are present, push the insulin back into the bottle quickly (this technique helps to get rid of the bubbles), and pull down slowly until you are at your *exact* insulin dose (when the plunger top is in line with the dose marker).**
9. **Repeat if necessary.**
10. **Take the needle out of the bottle and recap until you are ready to inject.**

they all have their own personality, right? Well, so does insulin! Keep this in mind as you read through the different classifications of insulin. Take time to look at your insulin's personality to see if it's right for you. If it's not, look at the other types of insulin to see if a different one might be a better match!

The different classifications of insulin include the rapid acting insulin called insulin analogs, which include Lispro (Humalog®) and Aspart (Novolog®); the short-acting regular insulin; the intermediate-acting types of insulin called Humulin®or Novulin® N or L (NPH or Lente); the long-acting insulin, Humulin® or Novulin® U (Ultralente); and the basal insulin analog called Lantus® (Glargine). Wow, a lot to choose from, right? Well, guess what? That's not all; there are different concentrations of insulin too!

The concentrations of insulin available in the United States are U-100 and U-500. This simply means there are 100 units of insulin per cc (cubic centimeter) or 500 units of insulin per cc. People who require large doses of insulin usually use U-500 insulin. But, most people in the United States use U-100 insulin. It's important for you to know that U-100 insulin is not available all over the world. So, you need to make sure you take extra supplies with you if and when you travel to a foreign country!

WHAT ARE THE DIFFERENT TYPES OF INSULIN?

Now let's talk about the different types of insulin. We'll start with regular insulin. This insulin is a clear liquid, so you can see through it. It's primarily used before a meal to cover the carbohydrate load or to correct a high blood glucose level. Regular insulin starts to work in about thirty to sixty minutes, and peaks (does most of its job) about two to four hours later. Generally speaking, regular insulin lasts for about six to twelve hours. So, if you take regular insulin before breakfast,

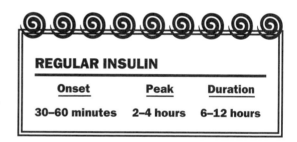

REGULAR INSULIN

Onset	Peak	Duration
30–60 minutes	2–4 hours	6–12 hours

you'll need to wait thirty to forty-five minutes before you have your breakfast. That's because you want your insulin to be doing most of its job about the same time that the food you eat turns to glucose and peaks in your blood. Are the management and monitoring requirements starting to make sense?

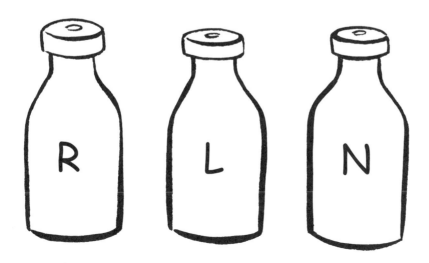

WHAT TO DO?

As mentioned before, sometimes regular insulin is also used to bring a high blood glucose down to the target level before a meal. When using regular insulin for this purpose, it's important to keep in mind the onset and peak time of action. Because, remember, regular insulin doesn't even start to work for at least thirty to sixty minutes, and it doesn't peak for about two to four hours. That means you'll need to give it time to work!

LET'S PRACTICE

$$320 \text{ mg/dl (before meal)}$$
$$- 120 \text{ mg/dl (your target)}$$
$$= 200 \text{ mg/dl (amount above target)}$$

In this scenario we can lower the blood glucose level 40 mg/dl for every unit of insulin taken.

200 mg/dl ÷ 40 mg/dl = 5 units needed to lower the blood glucose 200 mg/dl.

So, what do you do if your blood glucose is high before a meal? Well, here is an example. Let's say it's before dinner and your blood glucose level is 320 mg/dl. And let's say that according to the plan you and your healthcare professional worked out you are supposed to give yourself one unit of regular insulin for every 40 mg/dl you are above target. So, in other words if just before a meal your target is 120 mg/dl and you are at 320 mg/dl, you would need to give yourself five units of regular insulin just to get back to target. Now remember, that amount *doesn't* include what you would take to cover the carbohydrates in your meal. It's just the amount of insulin needed to get back to target (so that you can eat your meal without your blood glucose level going even higher). So now you can see why it's important to have a good understanding of what type of insulin you take and also how it works. That way you'll be able to anticipate what will happen with your blood glucose level after you've taken your insulin!

Okay, we've talked about regular insulin, now we need to talk about the insulin analogs (Lispro or Aspart), both of which are also clear liquids. If you notice particles, cloudiness, or discoloration of any type in clear insulin, it's no longer any good and it must be discarded. Or, if it's a new, unopened bottle of insulin it can be returned to the pharmacy. These types of insulin have a rapid onset once injected, so they start to work even faster than regular insulin does. Insulin analogs are also used to cover the carbohydrate load from a meal or to bring a high blood glucose level back to target level. However, Lispro and Aspart are different from regular insulin because they start to work very fast (about ten or fifteen minutes): they peak in about one to two hours and last for about three to six hours. This insulin really does have a different personality! As a result of this quick action, you don't have to wait for thirty minutes before you eat, just ten to fifteen minutes! Lispro and Aspart insulin are considered *dose and eat* types of insulin, so you'll need to make sure that you have some food available to eat before you take either of them!

INSULIN ANALOGS—LISPRO AND ASPART

Onset	Peak	Duration
10–15 minutes	1–2 hours	3–6 hours

Okay, let's say you're at a restaurant for dinner and you decide to take your Lispro or Aspart insulin when you get there, so you don't have to be bothered with it after you're seated. Is that a problem? It could be! If there were any delay in getting your food (like a waiting list, waiting for the waitress/waiter to take your order, or even a delay in the kitchen) that would be a problem because you already have insulin on board. That means that you would be putting yourself at risk for a low blood glucose reaction! Remember, you shouldn't wait any longer than ten to fifteen minutes to eat after you've taken either Lispro or Aspart insulin. What do you do about the restaurant scenario? Well, it would be better to give yourself insulin *after* you get your food (then go ahead and eat), rather than risk having low blood glucose.

Now let's talk about the types of insulin that are used to keep blood glucose levels at target in between meals. These types of insulin are referred to as intermediate, long-acting, or basal insulin depending on their onset, peak, and duration (more personalities). We'll begin with the intermediate acting types of insulin, NPH and Lente. NPH insulin is really just regular insulin with the addition of protamine and some zinc to make it last longer. So, instead of starting to work in thirty minutes, it starts to work in about one to two hours, peaks or does most of its job in about four to fourteen hours, and lasts

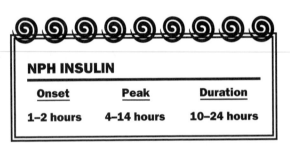

NPH INSULIN

Onset	Peak	Duration
1–2 hours	4–14 hours	10–24 hours

ten to twenty-four hours. Because we add a substance to regular insulin to make it last longer, it becomes cloudy. So this type of insulin will be milky white in color, but it shouldn't have any particles floating in it. Now in order to make sure this insulin works the same in the body each and every time you give it, you need to *resuspend* the insulin before drawing it up. That simply means you have to mix it first. The best way to mix insulin suspensions is to roll them or tip them from side-to-side twenty times. Yes, you heard me right, *twenty times*! If you do that consistently then you should get the same onset and peak each time you take it. And really, that's the key. You need to be able to reproduce the same response in blood glucose readings every single day. That doesn't mean you should get the same reading every day, it just means that you should be within a target range.

Lente insulin is also an intermediate type of insulin that has zinc added to it to make it last longer. Lente insulin's onset, peak, and duration are very similar to that of NPH. The color should be cloudy or milky white, so you can't see through this insulin, but there shouldn't be any particles in it. Because it is a solution, you'll need to resuspend it before using it, just like NPH. Again, this is done to make sure you are able to get that reproducible, consistent onset and peak. Now, unfortunately once you mix regular and Lente insulin, binding of the regular and Lente insulin begins, which changes the regular insulin. That's why it is recommended that the interval between mixing Lente and regular insulin and administering be the same each time you do it, so the results are always the same.

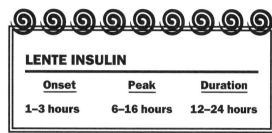

LENTE INSULIN

Onset	Peak	Duration
1–3 hours	6–16 hours	12–24 hours

When using these types of insulin in combination with fast acting regular or rapid acting Lispro or Aspart insulin, there is a sequence that must be followed in order to make sure that the clear rapid or fast acting insulin does not become contaminated. The main thing to remember is to always draw up the *clear* insulin first. Think about it. If you put a needle in a bottle of cloudy insulin (insulin suspension), the insulin touches the needle. Right? Yeah, it does. And a small amount remains in the needle because of the process of drawing it up into the syringe. If you were to put that needle into a bottle of clear insulin, you would contaminate it. So, the only way to prevent contamination when mixing two different types of insulin into one syringe is to always begin with the clear insulin first.

ULTRALENTE INSULIN

Onset	Peak	Duration
4–8 hours	10–30 hours	18–36 hours

That brings us to long-acting and basal insulin. These types of insulin are used for the same purpose as intermediate-acting insulin, which is to maintain blood glucose at target levels in between meals. Ultralente is a long-acting insulin suspension (regular insulin with more zinc added), so it doesn't start to work for four to eight hours (remember, you'll have to mix it). Ultralente insulin peaks in ten to thirty hours and can last for eighteen to thirty-six hours! Another insulin used to maintain blood glucose levels between meals is Glargine insulin (a.k.a. Lantus®). Glargine is a relatively new analog basal insulin that works a little differently from intermediate- and long-acting insulin. Glargine is not a suspension and it doesn't have a peak action; it's considered a *flat-acting* insulin. Once this insulin is maintained at a constant

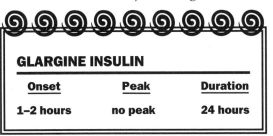

GLARGINE INSULIN

Onset	Peak	Duration
1–2 hours	no peak	24 hours

level in the blood, it remains relatively peakless. This means that if you continue to inject it at the same time every day, it will remain constant in the blood, and there will be no peaks and valleys. Now, as mentioned earlier, this medication is different because it is not a suspension. There isn't anything added to it to make it last longer, so it's clear. It's actually developed a little differently and it has a little different

INSULIN STORAGE GUIDELINES

- Store insulin in the refrigerator at 36° to 46° F (2° to 8° C).
- Store *unopened* insulin in the refrigerator until the expiration date on the package.
- You can store the insulin vial or cartridge you are currently using at room temperature to reduce local irritation at the injection site.
- Insulin vials can be stored at room temperature 59° to 86° F (15° to 30° C) for twenty-eight days, after that you have to throw the insulin out.
- Storage for insulin cartridges and pens are different based on the type of insulin.
- Lispro or regular insulin cartridges or prefilled pens may be kept at room temperature for twenty-eight days.
- 70/30 insulin cartridges or prefilled pens may be kept at room temperature for ten days.
- NPH cartridges or prefilled pens can be kept at room temperature for fourteen days.
- 75/25 insulin cartridges or prefilled pens may be kept at room temperature for ten days.
- Carry insulin and supplies with you when traveling (like in a carry-on bag); do not leave it in a car or put it in your airline luggage!

mechanism of action. An important precaution to remember about insulin Glargine is that you *can't* mix it with any other insulin. And because Glargine is clear, it could easily be confused with regular or rapid-acting insulin. You will notice, however, that the shape of the bottle is a little bit longer and the cap is purple, which is different from any other type of insulin currently on the market.

There are also combination types of insulin available. For example, 70/30 insulin is 70 percent NPH insulin mixed with 30 percent regular insulin. NPH and regular insulin can be mixed together and remain stable over time. Other combination insulins include 75/25 and Novolog® 70/30, which use NPL insulin in combination with Lispro or Aspart insulin. NPL insulin is really just another intermediate-acting insulin, very similar to NPH; it's just made with Lispro or Aspart insulin instead of regular insulin. With any of the combination types of insulin, it is very important to remember to resuspend the insulin correctly. Remember, you need to make sure that you get the same concentration of insulin each and every time, so that you can correctly predict your blood glucose outcome.

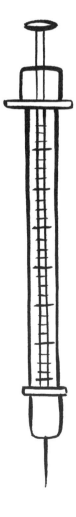

Now that you have a good idea of the different types of insulin available on the market, we need to discuss pattern management. There are a variety of different *recipes* that are used to maintain a person's glucose at target level. But, those recipes are really very individualized, based on things like your carb intake, exercise, stress in your life, and so on. For example, you know that you're going to need insulin to cover your meals and you'll also need insulin to cover your blood glucose in between meals. So, maybe you and your healthcare practitioner will decide on a management plan that includes an intermediate-acting insulin in the morning and a rapid- or fast-acting insulin (like Aspart, Lispro, or regular) before breakfast, lunch, and dinner, with an intermediate-acting insulin before bed. Or perhaps you would prefer taking a basal insulin once a day, such as Glargine, with injections of rapid-acting insulin to cover your carb intake. Sometimes, people even take regular insulin with an intermediate-acting insulin at breakfast, and

INSULIN ADMINISTRATION

1. **Choose your site. Make sure to rotate sites at least 1 inch from your last injection and no closer than 1½ inches from your belly button. Think of a way to remember where you need to give your next injection or write it down.**
2. **Clean the spot (soap and water works best, but you can use alcohol if soap and water aren't available).**
3. **Remove needle cap and hold syringe like a dart.**
4. **With your free hand pinch up some skin.**
5. **Stick the needle straight in (unless you are very thin, then use 45 degree angle), push in the plunger, and count to five before you remove the needle.**
6. **Discard your needle into a puncture proof container (hard plastic) or dispose of it according to your city or county regulations.**

take regular and an intermediate-acting insulin again at dinnertime. So you can see there are a variety of different recipes or patterns that can be used to manage your blood glucose levels over a period of time. It's just a matter of figuring out what works best for you based on your lifestyle and based on how you want to manage your diabetes.

There are even insulin pumps (discussed fully in chapter 10) available now. People using pumps are primarily using rapid-acting insulin (Lispro or Aspart) as part of their pump management. You see with a pump, tiny amounts of insulin are given all day and all night long. This is referred to as the *basal* insulin, which is very similar to the way your body would give you insulin naturally if it could, and what intermediate- or long-acting insulin does (via an insulin syringe) if you're not on the pump! Then a bolus of insulin is given just before a meal to cover the carb intake. This again is similar to what the body would do naturally if it could. Pump therapy is certainly another very viable alternative.

Regardless of what type of pattern management you choose, it's essential for you to recognize how important blood glucose monitoring is (so that you can see if what you

HELPFUL INSULIN TIPS

- The general rule is two insulins being mixed together should be from the same brand (i.e., Humulin® or Novolin®).
- Always draw up the regular, Lispro, or Aspart insulin first.
- Do not mix Glargine insulin with any other insulin!
- Syringes and needles can be reused if proper technique is used, but there may be a risk for infection in some people.
- You can inject insulin through clothes, but again there may be a risk for infection in some people.
- If you reuse syringes, safely recap the needle and store at room temperature (the needle may become dull with repeated use or the markings on the syringe may wear off, so be careful!).
- Always follow a specific routine for insulin injection including consistent technique, accurate dosage, and site rotation.
- Give insulin into the fat tissue—pick an area that you can grasp a fold of skin and inject at a 90 degree angle—thin people may need to pinch the skin and inject at a 45 degree angle.
- Rotate injection sites within one area of the body, then move to another area—allow a few weeks rest before returning to the original site, otherwise you could get a buildup of insulin, which can play havoc with your blood glucose levels.
- Injection sites include the abdomen (the fastest absorption site) followed by the arm, leg, and hip.

are doing is working). In addition, you'll need to know how your insulin works so you can make changes in your management plan based on the results of your detective work! Remember, this is all done in an effort to make your life easier. As crazzzzy as that sounds, it's true. Your life will not be easier with blood glucose levels bouncing all over! So the name of the game is diabetes self-management! Again, let your healthcare team review your blood glucose readings with you. Together make changes in timing, type, or amount of insulin best suited for you. With so many choices of insulin available, there's a combination just right for you!

TIPS FOR REMEMBERING TO ROTATE YOUR INSULIN SITES

1. Give injections on the left side of your body for the beginning of the month (days 1–15). For example, morning injection in the abdomen, evening injection in the thigh. There is enough area to give fifteen or sixteen injections 1 inch apart in each of these areas.
2. Then for the end of the month (days 16–30 or 31), give injections on the right side of your body!

That way you will always know where your injection goes based on the day of the month!

NOTES

1. Peter H. Chase, "'What Is Diabetes?' Understanding Insulin Dependent Diabetes" (2000), available at www.uchsc.edu/misc/diabetes/chap2.html (December 27, 2001).

2. Martha M. Funnell, Cheryl Hunt, Karmeen Kulkarni, Richard R. Rubin, and Peggy C. Yarborough, *A Core Curriculum for Diabetes Education* (Chicago: American Association of Diabetes Educators, 1998), 302.

3. Diabetes Forum, "The History of Diabetes," available at www.diabetesforum.net/eng_hist_life_after.htm (January 10, 2003).

4. Funnell et al., *A Core Curriculum for Diabetes Education*, 302.

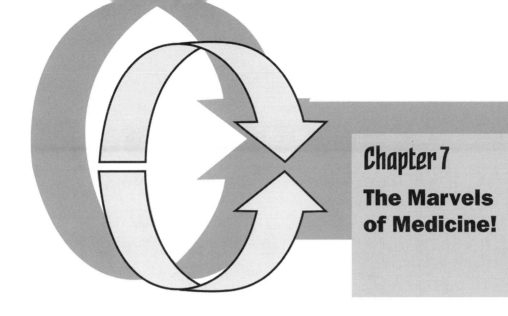

Chapter 7
The Marvels of Medicine!

You've probably already noticed that there's a lot of different stuff involved in managing diabetes. And for people with type 2 diabetes, oral medications may be a part of the diabetes plan. It's cool because there are several different types of medications out there now that can be used to help control blood glucose levels. For example, there are insulin secretion stimulators (tell the pancreas to make more insulin), insulin sensitizers (give the body cells an *attitude adjustment*, so insulin can do its job), and there are carbohydrate digestion delayers (work in the intestines, slowing down the absorption of carbohydrates so there's not a big rise in the

HOW DO INSULIN SECRETION STIMULATORS WORK?

◎ These medications stimulate your pancreas to make more insulin.

What are the different names of these types of medications?

Sulfonylureas
◎ Glucotrol® (glipizide)
◎ Micronase®, Diabeta®, Glynase® (glyburide)
◎ Amaryl® (glimepiride)

Meglidinides
◎ Prandin® (repaglinide)

D-phenylalanine derivatives
◎ Starlix® (nateglinide)

What's important to remember about these medications?

- Take sulfonylureas at the same time each day.
- Sulfonylureas may increase sensitivity to the sun—wear sun protection!
- Take Prandin® or Starlix® fifteen minutes before each meal—if you skip a meal you skip your Prandin® or Starlix®.
- Do not take other medications (including over-the-counter) without your doctor's okay.

---

blood glucose level after a meal). With all of these different medications, surely one of them will work for you if you have type 2 diabetes!

So how do all these medications work? Good question! Let's look at the insulin secretion stimulators first. In this group there are three main types of medications: The Sulfonylureas (yikes, what a name!), the Meglidinides (that name is not much better), and the D-phenylalanine deriviatives (makes ya wonder who thought up these great names).

As mentioned previously, the primary action of these drugs is to increase insulin production from the pancreas. That's why sometimes they're referred to as insulin secretagogues (insulin secretion stimulators). Because these medications cause the body to make more insulin, the major potential side effect is

---

What's are the potential side effects from these medications?

- Hypoglycemia
- Weight gain (from increased insulin secretion)
- Skin rash (rare)
- Upset stomach, diarrhea or constipation
- Upper respiratory infection (Prandin)
- Back discomfort (Prandin)
- Headache
- Dizziness

Who should not *take these medications?*

- Anyone with a known allergy to the medication.
- If you need surgery, have a trauma injury, or have a serious illness or infection, your doctor will probably take you off the medication until you recover.
- If you have kidney or liver disease or if you are malnourished, pregnant, or nursing, have type 1 diabetes, or have diabetic ketoacidosis, you should not take these medications (with the exception of Amaryl®, Starlix®, and Prandin®, which may be used in people with kidney impairment).

---

hypoglycemia (low blood glucose). See, if you were to take an insulin secretagogue and then let's say, forget to eat or skip a meal, you could have a low blood glucose reaction. So as far as these medications go, remember to eat according to your meal plan. If you take either Prandin® or Starlix®, remember to take your medication one to thirty minutes before you eat (fifteen minutes is a good halfway point), because these two medications are glucose dependent. That simply means that they begin to work as soon as glucose enters the blood, then the effects of the medication decrease as the glucose level in the blood declines. So, if you decide you're not going to eat a meal (by the way that's not a good idea), then don't take your Prandin® or Starlix®.

Now let's talk about the insulin sensitizers. These medications increase insulin sensitivity at the cell site, allowing insulin to do its job. Insulin sensitizers actually partially reverse the insulin resistance typically seen in type 2 diabetes!

HOW DO INSULIN SENSITIZERS WORK?

- These medications increase the insulin sensitivity at the cell site (kinda like a cell attitude adjustment!).
- Glucophage® also decreases glucose production in the liver.

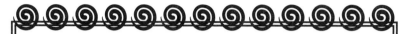

What are the different names of these types of medications?

Thiazolidinediones (TZDs)
- Actos® (pioglitazone)
- Avandia® (rosiglitazone)

Thiazolidinedione/Biguanide
- Avandamet® (combination of rosiglitazone and metformin)

Biguanides
- Glucophage® (metformin)

Biguanide/Sulfonylurea
- Glucovance® (combination of metformin and glyburide)
- Metaglip® (combination of metformin and glipizide)

In this group there are two main types of medications: the thiazolidinediones (yeah, the names keep getting worse and worse!) and the biguanides. And there are combination medications that include both of these types of medications: Avandamet® (combination of rosiglitazone and metformin), Glucovance® (combination of glyburide and metformin), and Metaglip® (combination of metformin and glipizide). So, the possibilities are literally unlimited!

There are a couple of important things to remember about these medications. First, you can expect your physician to evaluate your liver enzymes before you begin taking the medication and periodically after that, because in some people insulin sensitizers can cause liver problems. It's really pretty rare, but it still makes sense to have these blood tests done to make sure that your liver continues to function properly.

Second, drinking alcohol while taking Glucophage®

What's important to remember about these medications?

- Your physician will evaluate your liver enzymes.
- Drinking alcohol when taking Glucophage® increases the risk of lactic acidosis.
- Take Glucophage® with food to minimize side effects.

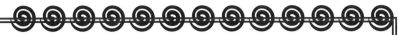

What are the potential side effects of insulin sensitizers?

Avandia® and Actos®
- Resumption of ovulation in women (risk of pregnancy)
- Potential for increased liver enzymes
- Anemia (Avandia®)
- Increased blood fats (Avandia®)

Glucophage®
- Some people complain of diarrhea, loss of appetite, upset stomach, and bloating initially.
- Lactic acidosis—a rare but serious condition. Symptoms include unexplained weakness, tiredness, dizziness, or trouble breathing.
- Slight weight loss.

Glucovance®
- Same as Sulfonylureas
- Same as Glucophage®

Avandamet®
- Same as Glucophage®
- Same as Avandia®

Metaglip®
- Same as Glucophage®
- Same as Sulfonylureas

Who should not take these medications?

Avandia® and Actos®
- Anyone with a history of liver disease, alcohol abuse, or cardiac problems.

Glucophage®
- History of kidney or liver disease
- History of lactic acidosis
- History of alcoholism or binge drinking
- This medication may be discontinued if you have kidney failure, have a heart attack, develop congestive heart failure, need surgery, or need tests that require iodinated contrast.

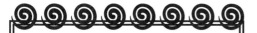

HOW DO CARBOHYDRATE DIGESTION DELAYERS WORK?

◎ These medications slow down the absorption of carbohydrates in the intestine. This causes the blood glucose level to go up slower and not as high after a meal.

increases the risk of lactic acidosis. This condition can occur when there is a build up of Glucophage® in the system. When the body is busy trying to get rid of the alcohol it can't metabolize the Glucophage® the way it is supposed to and it builds up in the blood. Lactic acidosis is very serious, sometimes even fatal! So, make sure you follow your physician's advice!

Next on the list are the carbohydrate digestion delayers. These medications work by slowing down the absorption of carbohydrates in the intestines. Because the glucose enters the blood at a slower rate, there is a gradual increase in blood glucose after a meal. This is ideal for people who tend to have high blood glucose one to two hours after eating.

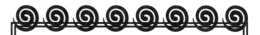

What are the different names of these types of medications?

Alpha-glucosidase Inhibitors
◎ Precose® (acarbose)
◎ Glyset® (miglitol)

The carbohydrate digestion delayers are also known as alpha-glucosidase inhibitors, which include Precose® (acarbose) and Glyset® (miglitol). These medications don't cause hypoglycemia when used alone. That's because they don't cause the body to

What are the potential side effects from these medications?

◎ Gas
◎ Abdominal discomfort
◎ Bloating
◎ Diarrhea
◎ Weight loss

(Side effects tend to occur when you first start taking these medications, then the symptoms diminish with time.)

make more insulin; they work by slowing down the glucose absorption. But, the important thing to remember about these medications is that if you take Precose® or Glyset® in combination with an insulin secretion

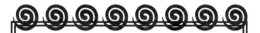

Who should not take these medications?

◎ Anyone with a known allergy to the medication or liver disease.
◎ Anyone with inflammatory bowel disease or other intestinal disorders.

stimulator, like Glucotrol®, Prandin®, Starlix®, or even insulin, you could have a low blood glucose episode. And if that does happen you have to treat it with glucose or lactose (the sugar found in milk), because alpha-glucosidase inhibitors slow down the absorption of sucrose (table sugar) or fructose (fruit or fruit juice) so they do not work.

Remember, you can't pop a pill and expect everything to be okay. It doesn't work that way. Oral medications work best when used in combination with meal planning and physical activity.

What's important to remember about these medications?

◎ Take with the *first bite* of the meal.
◎ Start with a low dose and build up slowly.
◎ These medications do not cause hypoglycemia when used alone, but if they are used in combination with insulin secretion stimulators, then hypoglycemia can occur. In this situation you will need to treat your hypoglycemia with glucose or lactose, like *glucose gel, glucose tablets,* or *skim milk.* Because these medications slow the breakdown of table sugar and fruit juices, these choices will not work.

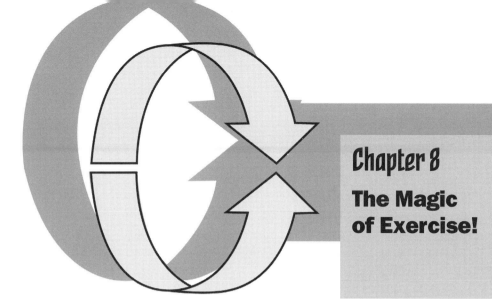

Chapter 8
The Magic of Exercise!

Did you know the benefits of physical activity can be traced all the way back to ancient times?! Wow, that means there must be some truth to what all those health nuts have been saying all along! And because of the great benefits of physical activity, it's considered a major player in diabetes management today.

Okay, so what's all the hype about? Let's talk about what happens in the body as a result of physical activity. When people with diabetes (especially people with type 2 diabetes) increase their physical activity level they use the insulin their body already makes a little better, so they may not need as much oral

PHYSICAL ACTIVITY IN ANCIENT TIMES

- Ancestors up through the beginning of the Industrial Revolution included strenuous physical activity as a normal part of their daily lives.
- Physical activity was seen as an important part of religious, social, and cultural expression.
- It was common for people to walk the 6- to 20-mile round-trip to visit other villages to see relatives and to trade with other clans.
- In India, proper diet and physical activity were known to be essential principles of daily living.
- Yoga, a philosophy that included a complicated series of stretching and flexibility postures, was identified as far back as 600 B.C.
- In ancient China, Tai chi chuan, an exercise system that teaches graceful movements, began as early as 200 B.C.[1]

medication or insulin in the form of injection.[2] Not only that, but if a person with diabetes continues on a physical activity plan over a period of time, he or she may notice improved insulin sensitivity, which allows the glucose in the blood to get into the cells easier. Certainly you've already heard about how great physical activity is for maintaining a healthy heart (physical activity helps to improve the functioning of the heart). People with diabetes have a higher risk of developing heart-related problems, so that's all the more reason to stay active!

Did you know. . . The average person walks around the earth 2-2.5 times in his or her lifetime!

AEROBICIZE!

Now, if you're not already *movin' and groovin'* in some form or another, you need to start thinking about what type of activity you enjoy. Keep in mind, most of the benefit from regular activity occurs when your body uses more oxygen to maintain the activity. This type of activity is often referred to as *aerobic*. Aerobic activity can include anything from biking, hiking, skating, dancing, to even just walking! When you include aerobic activity in your daily routine, it helps you stay at your desired body weight and it helps reduce A1c levels in people with type 2 diabetes (and even in some people with type 1 diabetes). Resistance exercise is another type of activity that can provide huge health benefits as well. Weightlifting is a good example of resistance exercise. This type of activity doesn't require increased oxygen to meet energy needs. When you lift weights you not only improve muscle strength, but you can also increase your endurance! So, whatever it is you like to do, just do it! Don't be the kind of person that just plays baseball on the computer! Get outside and really hit the ball!

PHYSICAL ACTIVITY AND HYPOGLYCEMIA

As you can probably guess, the immediate effects of physical activity generally cause a decrease in blood glucose levels. You already know that glucose is found in the blood after a carbohydrate meal and is stored in the liver and muscle cells in the form of glycogen. Your body also stores fat and amino acids (amino acids are the building blocks for all your cells). Now when you first start exercising, let's say the first thirty minutes or so, your body will use the glucose stored in your muscle cells. Then as you continue to exercise, your body will turn to the liver and fat tissues for energy. The body typically only uses amino acids as a last resort, only if nothing else is left. Hopefully, you'll never get to that point!

So you see, if you exercise and you don't replenish your body's main source of energy—glucose—you can develop hypoglycemia (low blood glucose). Hypoglycemia is considered the most common problem in people with diabetes that use insulin or other medications to lower blood glucose.[3] Part of this may be due to the fact that injected insulin is actually absorbed quickly during and/or after exercise. Or, sometimes a depot of insulin (stored in fat tissue from previous injections) is released during exercise, causing the blood glucose to drop. Another reason may be that the cells in the body become more sensitive to the insulin with increased activity (especially people with type 2 diabetes), so less insulin is needed to maintain the blood glucose level. Any way you look at it the result is basically the same, lower blood glucose.

POST-EXERCISE LATE-ONSET HYPOGLYCEMIA

Post-exercise late-onset (PEL) hypoglycemia is another phenomenon to watch out for. PEL is a low blood glucose that occurs four or more hours after exercise. Actually, PEL can even occur up to twenty-four hours after exercise! Generally speaking, this type of hypoglycemia happens more frequently in people with type 1 diabetes after moderate or high-intensity exercise that lasts for more than thirty minutes. This basically comes about as a result of what we talked about earlier. First, there may be increased insulin sensitivity, which causes more glucose to be used. Second, if the body uses glucose from storage areas during physical activity, then the glucose must be replaced (to restore the used stores for future use). As the body tries to refill those storage areas on its own, the blood glucose level continues to drop.

I like to play tennis, swim, rollerblade, and run. Sometimes I go low, but that's if I'm really pushing myself. Most of the time the activities help me stay level. —Nicole

Understand that in people without diabetes the pancreas is able to react very quickly when a person is exercising and helps the person out by decreasing the insulin that is being made. Even the liver helps out by producing more glucose for the body to use. As a result, the level of glucose in the blood stays about the same. In other words, the body makes up for the increase in sensitivity by making less insulin during and after physical activity in the person who doesn't have diabetes. But, when you have diabetes and you have to inject insulin into your body or take medication that makes your body produce more insulin, there is no way to *shut it off*. To make matters worse, the insulin that's already floating around tells the liver not to release stored glucose! Can you believe it! So the insulin causes the body to use up the glucose that's already available, but no additional glucose is released from the liver to make up for what is being used. This can truly cause a problem if you aren't aware of what to do to prevent this from happening in the first place.

EXERCISE AND HYPERGLYCEMIA (HIGH BLOOD GLUCOSE)

Well now, you think you've got it, right? Not so fast! Believe it or not, in some people (primarily in people with type 1 diabetes), the blood glucose can actually *increase* as a result of physical activity. You're probably thinking, "This is getting ridiculous! First the big concern is low blood glucose, now we're actually talking about the blood glucose level going too high after physical activity!" Gees, make up your mind! Right?

Well, the truth of the matter is physical activity of a high intensity can also cause blood glucose levels to go higher after the activity, even if the blood glucose level is normal to begin with. That's because when there isn't enough insulin in the body to allow the glucose to enter the cells, the body's counterregulatory hormones (adrenaline, cortisol, and so forth) increase and cause the liver to dump extra glucose in the blood, even though there is already plenty of glucose floating around!

Wait, there's still another situation that can cause the blood glucose level to rise as a result of physical activity. Remember, if the body can't use the glucose that's in the blood without insulin, it tries to find other ways to get fuel for energy. So, of course, the first thing it does is to try to release all stored glucose. After it does that, it tells the body to start breaking down fat. Now that's when the real trouble begins. Remember, if the body can't get rid of the byproduct of fat breakdown (ketones) fast enough, the ketones build up in the blood and make the person sick. But, again this is not the *primary* side effect of physical activity. Low blood glucose is! It's just important for you to know that hyperglycemia and/or ketosis can become worse after real intense physical activity that forces the body to look for alternative ways to get energy.

EXERCISE PRECAUTIONS

Okay, so now that you know what happens, what can you do about it? Well, glad you asked! There are a few special precautions for physical activity you should consider. First you need to keep in mind that your blood glucose level can be affected by the type, amount, and intensity of the activity. We really already discussed that, but what we didn't discuss is that blood glucose can also be affected by the timing and type of food

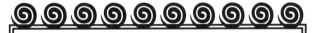

SAFETY FIRST!

1. Exercise after a meal (maybe wait an hour to give your body a chance to digest some food!).
2. Avoid late evening exercise due to risk of hypoglycemia when sleeping.
3. Carry some type of carbohydrate with you.
4. Check blood glucose before and after physical activity.
5. Wear diabetes identification.
6. Use proper equipment—like the right shoes!
7. Include a warm-up and cool-down.
8. Drink plenty of fluids.
9. If it's really hot, humid, or even cold out, avoid an extreme workout.

you had at your last meal. So let's say you have a nice salad for lunch and then you decide to go out and run a couple of miles an hour later. Problem! Not enough carb to sustain the activity! Duh!

So, after hearing all of that you're probably thinking, why bother? There's too much to think about. Hey, don't sweat the small stuff; remember it's all small stuff! These things can easily be managed with a little planning and thinking ahead. In other words, you need to follow the *guidelines for physical activity*.

No joke, really, there are guidelines for what some people call exercise, but what others who are really *in the know* call physical activity. This isn't rocket science; it's just plain old common sense. First, meet with your healthcare professional and work out an activity plan. After talking with your healthcare professional you may decide that you can keep your blood glucose in control best by decreasing your medication or short-acting insulin. Some people decide to decrease their total daily insulin only during the time of physical activity. Still others decide to wait and participate in physical activity 2 or 3 hours after a meal in order to keep their blood glucose in control and prevent hypoglycemia. Don't worry; you'll be able to decide what will work best for you once you talk with your healthcare professional! Second, check your blood glucose before you begin any change in activity. You know, like maybe today you decide you want to be a marathon runner! Well, it might be a good idea if you check your blood glucose first! You wouldn't go fishing without a fishing pole would ya?

Oh, another important thing to remember is not to give your insulin injection in a muscle by mistake. Because muscle contractions may increase the absorption of insulin in the blood, it is essential that you give your insulin injection in the fat tissue, where it is supposed to be given. So again, remember to check your blood glucose level before and even after you exercise until you know how your blood glucose is likely to

Remember. . . make good choices to keep your health tipped in your favor!

I'm in the marching band. This affects my blood glucose levels a lot, because I play the biggest drum in the band. It helps me get more exercise in my arms.
—Everett

respond. That way you will be able to determine if you'll need to adjust your insulin and/or carb intake with that particular physical activity.

We didn't really talk about carb intake yet, did we? Yes, yet another choice that you have is to increase your carb intake to cover physical activity. For example, sometimes people will add carbs when they have unplanned activity or when they're participating in physical activity for an extended period of time. You know, like the marathon runner! Now, the amount of carbohydrates you'll need to eat depends on a couple of things as well. Once again, you need to consider the time of the exercise in relation to when you took your insulin (you have to know when your insulin is going to peak) or your medication, when you ate last, the type and duration of activity, and what your blood glucose level was before you started.[4] So that's another reason why it's important to learn as much as you can about *your* diabetes and work with a healthcare professional who can help

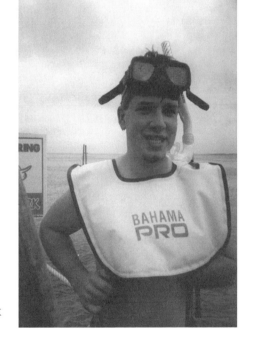

you sort all this stuff out. Just like everything else we've discussed so far, physical activity must be individualized for you. That's right, based on what your preference is, your physical fitness level, and your schedule.

ACTIVITY THAT'S RIGHT FOR YOU!

Not everyone loves sports or is destined to be a marathon runner, but you can find the best activities for your life. There are lots of cool things out there to help everyone keep active! No matter what your style is, you need to get out there and move. A good goal for teens is at least thirty minutes of activity per day, on most if not all days! Remember, though, you really need to talk about this plan with your healthcare professional first!

> **I play hockey for Eastern Michigan University. Activity usually causes my blood glucose level to go up . . . but I wear an insulin pump to control my blood glucose level.**
> **—Steven**

So what's your style? Are you an *avid athletic*? If so, you probably really like to compete, right? Maybe your big dream is to play in the NFL? Or maybe you visualize yourself playing

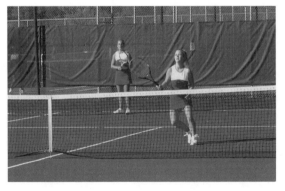

basketball with Michael Jordan. Well, that's possible, but the best thing for you to keep in mind is *everything in moderation*! And, try finding some things you like to do by yourself, too. Maybe biking or swimming, that way when you're *over-the-hill* (like twenty-five!), you'll still be able to enjoy some type of physical activity that doesn't require beating up your body!

If you're a *bona fide teen* and you're always busy having fun, the best thing for you to keep in mind is to always work in some type of *fun* that will help keep your body in shape. For example, maybe you'd like to try white-water rafting (yeah, right!) or just plain old running. That way you get more for your money, fun, and fitness too!

Don't fret if your style is *simple solitude*. Maybe you like being active but you prefer to do it alone? Well, there are plenty of cool suggestions for you, too! Just think of Tour de France winner Lance Armstrong! But remember, you can spice up your life by trying some team sports and make new friends to boot.

Okay, so what if you don't fit into any of these styles. No sweat! (No pun intended!) There's stuff for you to do too! Let's say you don't participate in any extra physical activity because you're just too darn busy! Sound familiar? Maybe you're the type that's out and about 24/7? Well, the best way to get into the activity loop is to use some of your social charm to get you and your friends physically fit. You'll make time to be with your friends, right? Cool, so maybe you could walk at the mall instead of just hanging out, or maybe suggest a social gathering that involves swimming, softball, or even some golf (of course you'll need to walk the course, not ride)!

If you're thinking this exercise stuff doesn't sound like any fun, the problem is the way you're thinking about it. Yeah, that's it! You just

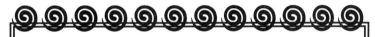

CHECK IT OUT!

www.health.org
www.diabetes-exercise.org
www.surgeongeneral.gov/sgoffice.htm
www.joslin.harvard.edu/education/libra
www.jdrf.org/
www.niddk.nih.gov/
www.diabetes.org/education/exercise/FAQs.htm

need an attitude adjustment! Remember we're just talking about physical activity here, not the old if there's *no pain, there's no gain* adage. Just get out and move, put the PS2 down, shut off the computer, and get out of that chair! Besides the benefits from blood glucose control and cardiovascular health, you can also reap a lot of rewards in terms of psychological health from activity as well. For example, people who are physically active feel they have a better quality of life than those who aren't active. It can also help you decrease stress. So, if you want to be more in control of your life and of your diabetes, get *movin*'!

NOTES

1. Centers for Disease Control (CDC), "Historical Background and Evolution of Physical Activity Recommendations," available at www.cdc.gov/nccdphp/sgr/intro2.htm (November 21, 2002).

2. Marion J. Franz, Karmeen Kulkarni, William H. Polonsky, Peggy Yarborough, and Virginia Zamudio, *A Core Curriculum for Diabetes Education: Diabetes Management Therapies* (Chicago: American Association of Diabetes Educators, 2001), 58.

3. Martha M. Funnell, Cheryl Hunt, Karmeen Kulkarni, Richard R. Rubin, and Peggy C. Yarborough, *A Core Curriculum for Diabetes Education* (Chicago: American Association of Diabetes Educators, 1998), 262.

4. Funnell et al., *A Core Curriculum for Diabetes Education*, 267.

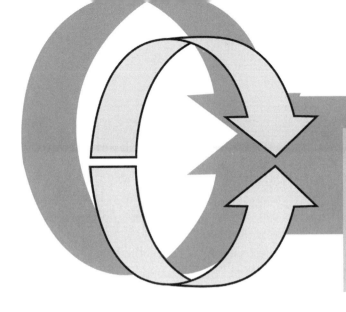

Chapter 9
Let Me Off This Roller Coaster!

Have you ever had one of those days, or weeks, or months when your blood glucose level goes up, then down, then up again? Have you ever just wanted to have a day of consistent blood glucose readings? Well, good news! The day has arrived and you, my friend, can be the captain of the ship! We're talking about blood glucose control through pattern management, of course. Just think, you can actually use all the information you gather on a daily basis to help you obtain your glucose goals! Yeah! There's truly a good reason for writing down all those numbers! So if you're ready to get off the roller coaster, hang on, here we go!

> When your blood glucose is out of control and you never do anything about it, your eyesight can go bad, you can end up with some heart problems, and even end up getting a body part amputated. —Steve

First, remember how we went through all that insulin and medication stuff earlier? You learned about how insulin and oral diabetes medications work, and about preparing and administering insulin. Well, that's a real important part of pattern management because you have to know how your medication and/or insulin works in order to determine how it will affect your blood glucose level. That's why it's so important for you to get into diabetes education classes and learn as much as you can about diabetes management. But, that's not all; you also have to be willing to check your blood glucose at specific intervals, to count carbohydrates (accurately!), to keep physically active pretty consistently, and to keep good records.

Keeping records?! What a pain in the butt!

Yeah, it's a pain, but you need to record what's happening on a daily basis in order to be able to identify trends. There are some monitors out on the market now that can do that for you. There are even some Personal Digital Assistant programs available to help as well!

Keep your blood glucose in balance. . .

Let's talk a little bit about what it means to identify trends. Well, let's say that your blood glucose level has been staying within your target goals (remember these are *your* goals) and you leave for a vacation in Spain. You're eating new foods, trying different dishes, and eating at different times of the day. By the end of the third day you notice that your blood glucose levels have been slowly creeping upward, especially after meals. What do you think is going on? Well, why don't you try to guess the most likely reason for the change in the blood glucose level and write it down? What do you think is the cause? You guessed it! One of the reasons this could be happening may be due to inaccurately estimating the carbohydrate content in the new (and exciting) foods that you've been eating. Eating new food is not a bad thing! Variety is the spice of life! But you may not notice that the change in blood glucose is related to the food you're eating unless you keep good records. So, in this case, you've done good detective work; now you just need to become familiar with the amount of carbohydrates that's in the food that you're trying. Maybe you could buy a book of Spanish cuisine that indicates carbohydrate grams per serving.

You might even go back to weighing and measuring your food for a few days until you become accustomed to the types of foods available and how they affect your blood glucose level.

PATTERN MANAGEMENT TAKES COMMITMENT!

Pattern management can be a great way of controlling your blood glucose level, but it does take commitment on your part. It really helps if you have a support team that you can go to for help when needed. Maybe you could enlist your parents, a few good friends, your doctor, dietitian, and certified diabetes educator to start. Pattern management includes looking at your blood glucose levels and making adjustments in your management based on the patterns that you identify. The key is to keep your blood glucose level within your target level most of the time, so that you can prevent those irritating high and low blood glucose symptoms. It becomes very frustrating to continually chase high blood glucose readings with insulin, doesn't it? Just remember to look at the big picture: your physical activity level, carb intake, and medication to make sure all are in balance so that you don't end up falling off the boat! Here's a little guide to help keep you on course!

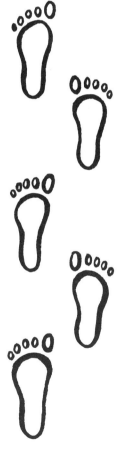

HOW CAN I GET A GRIP ON PATTERN MANAGEMENT?

This pattern management stuff really comes down to how you want to live with *your* diabetes. That means the final decisions regarding what you will do rest on you. This is *your* right, but it is also *your* responsibility. That's because you are the expert in *your* diabetes! Sure you will need guidance from healthcare professionals, but when it comes right down to it no one knows your life better than you. That means you are the one with all the power. So, use the power wisely. Learn how to take positive approaches to diabetes-related situations by making *informed* decisions. Use coping skills that protect you from slipping into self-care that is not productive. Surround yourself with people who have knowledge and skills about diabetes and who can help you make the best decisions for you!

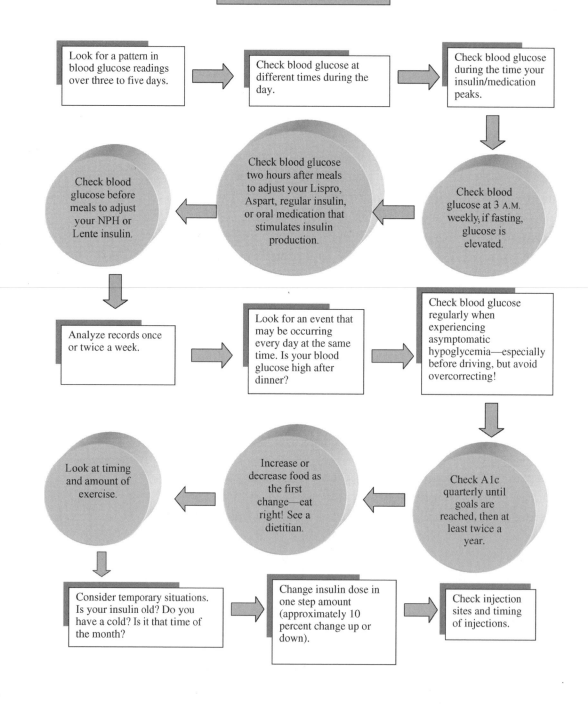

Pattern Management Flow Chart

Look for a pattern in blood glucose readings over three to five days.

Check blood glucose at different times during the day.

Check blood glucose during the time your insulin/medication peaks.

Check blood glucose before meals to adjust your NPH or Lente insulin.

Check blood glucose two hours after meals to adjust your Lispro, Aspart, regular insulin, or oral medication that stimulates insulin production.

Check blood glucose at 3 A.M. weekly, if fasting, glucose is elevated.

Analyze records once or twice a week.

Look for an event that may be occurring every day at the same time. Is your blood glucose high after dinner?

Check blood glucose regularly when experiencing asymptomatic hypoglycemia—especially before driving, but avoid overcorrecting!

Look at timing and amount of exercise.

Increase or decrease food as the first change—eat right! See a dietitian.

Check A1c quarterly until goals are reached, then at least twice a year.

Consider temporary situations. Is your insulin old? Do you have a cold? Is it that time of the month?

Change insulin dose in one step amount (approximately 10 percent change up or down).

Check injection sites and timing of injections.

Remember also that you are a physical, emotional, social, and spiritual person. As a result, your pattern management will involve looking at the big picture. What that means is, just like a weekend of dietary indulgences can affect your blood glucose, so can a glum spirit. All of the different aspects of your life are interrelated and must be taken into account when you make your diabetes management decisions. So, think about what is on your agenda and go with it!

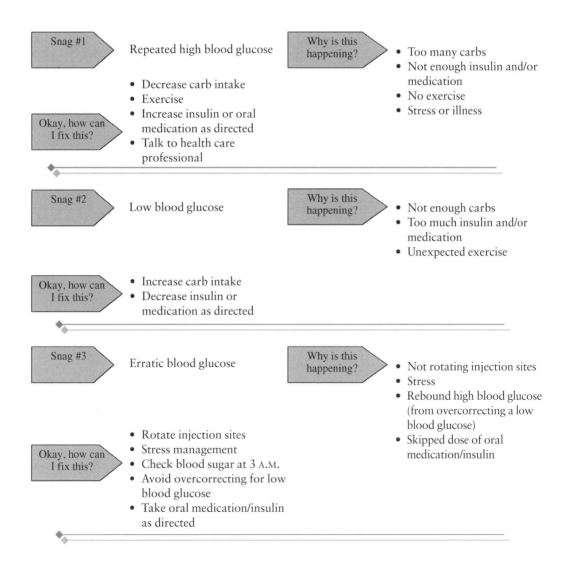

Snag #1 — Repeated high blood glucose

Why is this happening?
- Too many carbs
- Not enough insulin and/or medication
- No exercise
- Stress or illness

Okay, how can I fix this?
- Decrease carb intake
- Exercise
- Increase insulin or oral medication as directed
- Talk to health care professional

Snag #2 — Low blood glucose

Why is this happening?
- Not enough carbs
- Too much insulin and/or medication
- Unexpected exercise

Okay, how can I fix this?
- Increase carb intake
- Decrease insulin or medication as directed

Snag #3 — Erratic blood glucose

Why is this happening?
- Not rotating injection sites
- Stress
- Rebound high blood glucose (from overcorrecting a low blood glucose)
- Skipped dose of oral medication/insulin

Okay, how can I fix this?
- Rotate injection sites
- Stress management
- Check blood sugar at 3 A.M.
- Avoid overcorrecting for low blood glucose
- Take oral medication/insulin as directed

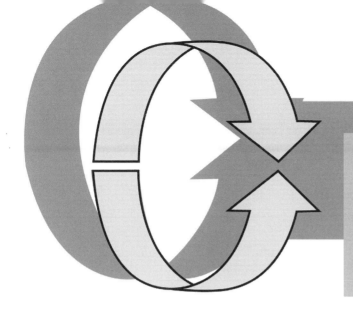

Chapter 10
The Freedom of Pumping!

Have you heard about insulin pumps or continuous insulin infusion (CSII) devices? These devices are like little computers that deliver insulin under the skin through a tiny catheter. This method of insulin delivery is promoted as a more physiological pattern of insulin delivery than what is currently being achieved through multiple injections of insulin. See, a person without diabetes has insulin that is released in little spurts throughout the day. The insulin is released according to the food that is eaten, activity that occurs, or hormones that are in the blood (some hormones cause the blood glucose level to go up). Insulin that's

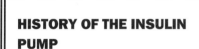

HISTORY OF THE INSULIN PUMP

◉ The first insulin pump also delivered glucagon. This pump was developed in the late 1970s at Whitehall Laboratories (Anacin) in Elkhart, Indiana.

◉ It was so large it had to be worn on a person's back! Wow, things have really changed over the years!

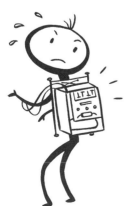

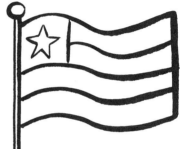

released in between meals or at night is referred to as *basal* or background insulin. It just keeps the blood glucose at an even level throughout the day and night. The insulin that's released when the person eats is called the *bolus* insulin. That insulin is used to cover the rise in blood glucose level after a meal. The insulin pump works in a similar manner. The pump can be programmed to deliver basal insulin throughout the day and night. Then when you eat, you simply give yourself a bolus of insulin by pushing a button on the pump to cover the anticipated rise in your blood glucose level after the meal.

HOW DOES THE INSULIN PUMP WORK?

The insulin pump is a battery-operated device that is designed to deliver rapid or fast-acting insulin (these are the only types of insulin that can be used in a pump) in programmed amounts throughout the day. The pump is 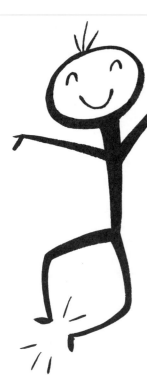 about the size of a pager, so it can be worn very discreetly under the clothes, on your belt, or in a pocket. The insulin is stored in a container, similar to an insulin syringe, only fatter and large enough to hold several days worth of insulin. The insulin is delivered through a small plastic tube that is attached to your body by using a cannula (an even smaller plastic tubing). You insert the cannula, with the help of a needle, into the fat tissue. Then the needle is removed, leaving the cannula in place. The cannula is changed every two to three days.

The goal of pump therapy is to imitate, as closely as possible, what the body would do normally if it could. So, a basal dose is programmed into the pump to keep the blood glucose level stable in between meals and during the night. This simply means the pump gives you little blurbs of insulin all day and all night long to keep the blood glucose within the target range. The amount of insulin that is programmed into the pump is based on your blood glucose results. For this reason, it's important for you to monitor your blood glucose level frequently and to keep accurate records (there's that word again). When you eat, you inject a bolus of insulin by pushing a button on the pump (like the rapid acting insulin some people take before meals with a syringe). Again, the purpose of the bolus is to cover the amount of carbohydrates you will eat with the meal or snack and/or to correct a high blood glucose level before eating. The physician and/or diabetes educator can help you work out the proper basal and bolus rates and help you adjust these rates as necessary. Eventually, there will be a pump available that'll be able to check your blood glucose level and give you insulin based on the results. Won't that be great?!

THE BENEFITS OF PUMPING

There are many benefits to using an insulin pump. First of all, the insulin pump can help you reach your target goals. Because the pump delivers tiny blurbs of insulin all day long, the absorption of the insulin tends to be more reliable. It can also increase your flexibility. For example, you no longer have to time your meals according to your insulin peaks; you can eat when you're hungry! So, meals really can be eaten at any time, as long as you bolus for your carb intake. Also, you can give yourself insulin anywhere you happen to be, and nobody else has to know about it! Insulin pump therapy means you can sleep in if you want to, and you can adjust your insulin easily for any change in activity.

If you're worried about what people will think if they see you wearing a pump, or if you're afraid your friends will make fun of you, hey, no sweat! No one has to know. You really can put this thing in places that no one will ever know! Or, if you're worried that the pump will come unattached or pull out during activity, there are precautions you can take to prevent this from happening as well. For example, you can reinforce the pump site with tape or even disconnect the pump during contact sports or rough activity. So see, there's a way around just about any potential problem!

ARE THERE RISKS WITH PUMPING?

Are there risks associated with pump therapy? Sure. But remember there are risks involved when you cross the street, when you get in a car, or even when you take insulin using a syringe. The key is to be prepared! So, what types of risks are we talking about? Well, basically high or low blood glucose. For instance, if the tubing on the pump is crimped or becomes dislodged, then no insulin is delivered to your body. So, if this happens and you don't recognize it, there is a risk of developing severe high blood glucose or even ketoacidosis. However, pump manufacturers have addressed this problem. Currently, all pumps on the market are equipped with alarms to alert you when a problem with the pump occurs. However, you must check your blood glucose level at specific intervals to identify a potential problem early, because the first sign of a problem may be high blood glucose. And once again, that's where your strong detective skills will come into play! The high blood glucose level may be due to sickness, stress, or even eating too many carbs for the amount of insulin that you bolused. In these circumstances you may need to adjust your pump basal and/or bolus rates to compensate for the situation. Some people even get high blood glucose from an infection at the insertion site. That's why it's important to change the infusion site every two or three days and change the tubing as instructed by the manufacturer.

Low blood glucose can also be a risk associated with pump therapy or any insulin therapy that involves intensive management. It's interesting, though, some people actually go on pump therapy to help reduce the frequency of low blood glucose events that occur with intensive therapy using an intermediate- and short-acting insulin. So really, low blood glucose is just one more reason why it's important to monitor your blood glucose regularly and to make necessary adjustments.

WILL WEARING A PUMP INTERFERE WITH MY LIFE?

Are you worried that pump therapy will interfere with your life? Well, if you are, you can stop worrying. Pump therapy won't interfere with your life if you don't let it! It usually takes three to six months to become completely comfortable wearing a pump. During this time your blood glucose levels will even out and you'll become accustomed to wearing it. And remember, you're not in this alone. Your healthcare professional, dietitian, or certified diabetes educator will be able to give you valuable information and guidance in managing your diabetes using pump therapy. And don't be afraid to enlist the help of family or friends. That's what they are there for! But, just like anything else that's new in your life, it does take some getting used to. So, cut yourself some slack. Expect that there will be a transition period, and most of all *keep an open mind*.

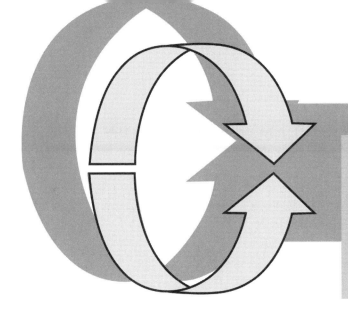

Chapter 11

I'm Sick with the Flu, What Do I Do?

Illness can certainly cause your blood glucose level to go up or down or just plain out of whack! Typically, blood glucose levels go up when a person is sick because of the release of stress hormones in the blood during illness or any kind of stress. See, when the body doesn't have enough fuel for energy or if it can't use the glucose that's already floating around in the blood because of a lack of working insulin, it dumps extra glucose in the blood that's stored in the liver. So your blood glucose level keeps going up and up. Eventually your body tries to get rid of the glucose in your blood by pulling fluid from the cells to make extra urine to flush the glucose out of the body. However, if the blood glucose level isn't corrected, this can lead to dehydration.

That's why it's important for you to follow a plan whenever you're sick, because if you become dehydrated and ketones start to build up in the blood, then the real trouble begins—you guessed it, ketoacidosis. This condition is more likely to develop in people with type 1 diabetes; however, ketoacidosis can occur in people with type 2 diabetes as well. Illness, infection, stress, injury, or even not enough insulin or oral diabetes medication (you know, like if you accidentally forget to take it) can bring on diabetic ketoacidosis (DKA).

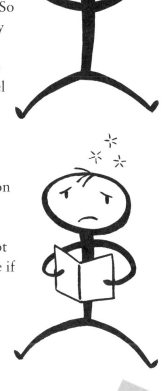

> When I had ketoacidosis I was totally oblivious to the state I was in.—Everett

SO WHAT IS DIABETIC KETOACIDOSIS?

Diabetic ketoacidosis is a metabolic acidotic state that occurs as a result of a lack of working insulin coupled with dehydration. Remember, if your body can't use the glucose that's in the blood because there's not enough insulin or because the insulin that's there doesn't work very well, it starts to look around for another source of energy. It begins to break down fat very rapidly to use as an alternative source of energy, causing an accumulation of ketones (the byproduct of fat metabolism). The body freaks out more when it realizes that there's all this glucose in the blood that it can't use because there's not enough working insulin. So it pulls fluids from the cells in an attempt to make extra urine to flush the glucose out of the blood. Now if you don't drink enough fluids to replace what your body is pulling out of your cells, you will become dehydrated. This stresses your body out even more, causing the release of stress hormones like cortisol and adrenaline. These hormones cause your body to release stored glucose from your liver to make it available for your brain, and to make matters worse, they make the insulin that is available less effective!

SIGNS OF DIABETIC KETOACIDOSIS

- High blood glucose—ketones in urine/blood
- Feeling sick to your stomach
- Vomiting
- Lack of appetite
- Dry, flushed skin
- Fruity odor to your breath
- Difficulty breathing
- Feel very weak
- Very thirsty
- Frequent urination

WHEN IS DIABETIC KETOACIDOSIS MORE LIKELY TO OCCUR?

- During illnesses like the flu.
- After an injury, like an infected cut.
- Even from not taking your insulin; remember if you're sick, even if you don't feel like eating, you still need insulin!
- Sometimes people who wear an insulin pump can develop DKA from plugged tubing, which prevents insulin from coming through the pump.

HOW IS KETOACIDOSIS TREATED?

So how is ketoacidosis treated? Well, the best treatment is prevention. Know what your blood glucose level is, and if it's over 250 mg/dl, check for ketones in your urine or blood (some monitors now have the capacity to check for ketones in the blood as well). Follow your healthcare practitioner's advice for treating ketones. Trace or small ketones in the urine can usually be cleared effectively by drinking plenty of calorie-free fluids. But, if you have moderate to large amounts of ketones in your urine, you will require medical assistance, extra fluids, and insulin (even if you don't usually use insulin), so make sure to call your healthcare practitioner!

Remember, a person with diabetes that develops ketoacidosis becomes ill very quickly. It's a dangerous condition that needs immediate attention. Once moderate ketoacidosis develops, especially with vomiting, the person may be hospitalized and started on fluids and insulin through a vein. During this time the person is watched closely because changes in the body chemicals can occur rapidly, making the person even sicker. So, now you can see why it's very important to get medical attention quickly if you start to develop signs of ketoacidosis!

SO, IF I'M SICK, WHAT DO I DO? . . . FOLLOW SICK-DAY GUIDELINES

1. Check your blood glucose more frequently when you feel sick—sometimes the first sign of illness is high blood glucose. Your blood glucose can reach into the 200s, 300s, or even 400s while you're sick.

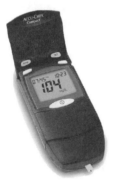

Accu-Chek Compact meter courtesy of Roche Diagnostics

2. Check your urine for ketones when your blood glucose is over 250 mg/dl. Ketones build up more frequently in people with type 1 diabetes, but can occur in people with type 2 as well.

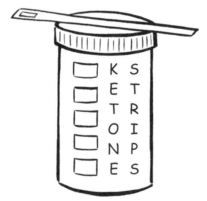

3. Call your health care professional for instructions if your blood glucose remains over 250 mg/dl or below 60 mg/dl, or if you have moderate or large ketones in your urine. You should also call your healthcare professional if you're not feeling better in two days, or if you continue to have diarrhea or vomit for more than six hours.
4. Continue taking your medication when you're sick (unless instructed otherwise from your physician), even if you are unable to eat. Remember, hormones are released during stress and illness that can make your blood glucose level even higher.

(*continued*)

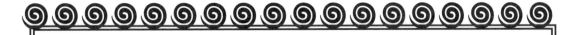

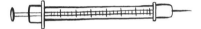

5. Sometimes additional doses of rapid-acting insulin may be needed (even if you normally just use oral medication to manage your diabetes).

6. Make sure you continue taking in fluids so that you don't become dehydrated. Drink plenty of calorie-free, caffeine-free liquids (caffeine causes more fluid loss) while you're awake; maybe some water, broth, or a sugar-free soft drink. When you're vomiting, have diarrhea, or have high blood glucose, your body loses extra fluid, which can lead to dehydration if you don't do anything about it. That's why it's important to replace the fluid you're losing. Fluids also help to flush the extra glucose and ketones out of the body.

7. If you can't stomach solid foods, then try clear liquids. It's best to stay on your regular meal plan when sick, but sometimes that's just not possible! So, try to take in about 15 grams of carbohydrates every hour or so to replace the food you normally would have eaten.

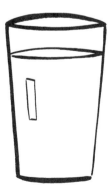

FOODS WITH 15 GRAMS OF CARBOHYDRATES . . .

- 6 saltine crackers
- 1 cup of chicken soup
- 1 slice of toast
- ½ cup cooked cereal
- ½ cup mashed potatoes
- ½ cup fruit juice
- 4 oz. regular soft drink
- 3 graham crackers
- ½ cup of regular Jello®

The American Diabetes Association recommends that everyone older than six months who has diabetes get a yearly flu vaccine and a onetime pneumococcal vaccine.

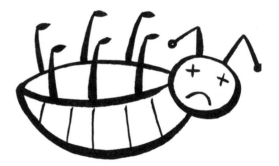

REMEMBER! PREVENTION IS THE KEY!

- Check your blood glucose level frequently when you are ill or have an infection, stress, or injury.
- Check your urine or blood for ketones when your blood glucose level is over 250 mg/dl.
- Do not exercise if you have ketones—exercise will cause more stress on your body.
- Drink plenty of calorie-free liquids.
- Call your healthcare professional for support.
- Take your insulin or oral medication as directed, even if you can't eat!
- Get plenty of rest, and take care of yourself!

"SICK DAY BOX" CHECKLIST

- calorie-free fluid choices
- crackers
- can of chicken noodle soup
- can of regular ginger ale
- box of regular Jello®
- ketone strips
- thermometer
- physician's telephone number

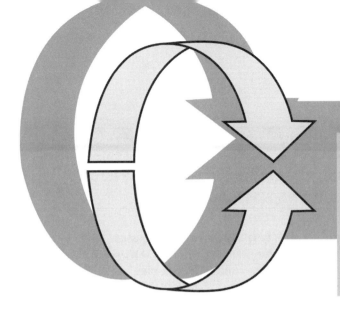

The Good News! You Have Control Over the Complications of Diabetes!

There's no doubt you've heard about the possible complications of diabetes. Things like heart and kidney disease, blindness, or even amputations. While it's true that some people develop complications from diabetes (even during the teen years), the good news is you can do something about it! Research results from the Diabetes Control and Complications Trial (DCCT) proved that maintaining blood glucose control over time helps to prevent or delay the onset of complications.[1] So, keep in mind as you are reading about the potential complications of diabetes that you are still *in control*. There are a lot of things you can do to stay healthy! Just because you have diabetes doesn't mean that these complications are inevitable! That's why the focus of this chapter is the *good news*! So if you think you're ready, hang on, here we go!

The Good News!

> ### DIABETES CONTROL AND COMPLICATIONS TRIAL (DCCT)
>
> - 1983–1993
> - 1441 people with type 1 diabetes participated.
> - Involved twenty-nine clinical centers in the United States and Canada, and eight central laboratories and units participated in the trial.
> - Showed that tight control of blood glucose levels can decrease and/or prevent the complications of diabetes.
> - Tight control included: Testing blood glucose levels four or more times a day; four daily insulin injections or use of an insulin pump; adjustment of insulin doses according to food intake and exercise; a diet and exercise plan; monthly visits to a healthcare team composed of a physician, nurse educator, dietitian, and behavioral therapist.[2]

WHAT ARE THE RISK FACTORS?

The complications of diabetes can be categorized into two primary groups: macrovascular (involving the large blood vessels in the body that lead to heart disease, strokes, and disease of the arms, legs, and feet) and microvascular disease (involving the small blood vessels in the body that lead to kidney disease or blindness). But before we begin, we need to talk about what situations or circumstances put a person at greater risk for developing complications from diabetes. In other words, modifiable (changeable) and nonmodifiable (nonchangeable) risk factors.

Duration of Diabetes and Age

So, what's a nonmodifiable risk factor? Good question. Nonmodifiable risk factors are those things that you really have no control over. For example, nonmodifiable risk factors include things like the genes you inherit, how long you've had diabetes, your gender, race, or even your age.

For instance, the longer a person has type 1 diabetes the more risk that person has for developing heart and kidney disease. But keep in mind this is also true for age in general. The older a person is the more chance he or she has for developing heart disease.

Genetics and Gender

As we mentioned previously, genetics and gender play a role as well. For example, men without diabetes have a greater chance of developing heart disease than women (before menopause) without diabetes. But, when diabetes is thrown into the mixture, women and men are suddenly at equal risk. That's because women lose their gender protective advantage once they develop diabetes.

Race

Okay, how about race? Well, race is also a risk factor for heart disease for some people with diabetes. For example, African Americans are at increased risk for developing macrovascular disease (involves the large blood vessels of the body), which includes heart disease, but have a lower chance of having an actual heart attack than Caucasians with diabetes.[3] Similarly, Mexican Americans are also at decreased risk for having a heart attack, but have an increased risk for peripheral vascular disease (involves the blood vessels in your hands and feet). So you can see how your age, race, or how long you've had diabetes may affect your risk for developing complications.

CONTROL MODIFIABLE RISK FACTORS!

So far we've been talking about all of those things in life that you really have no control over or really can't change. But there are some things that you do have control over, and these are called modifiable risk factors. These are the things that you can change! In other words, you have control! Okay, so what are modifiable risk factors? Well, modifiable risk factors are things like high blood glucose, high blood pressure, high cholesterol, smoking, obesity, and lack of activity (you know, the old couch potato syndrome!).

Blood Glucose

High blood glucose from poorly controlled diabetes can lead to conditions that damage the body's nerves and/or damage the blood vessels of the heart, kidneys, or even the eyes. So the closer you can keep your blood glucose level to your target goal, the better chance you will have of preventing these complications from ever developing. This seems logical right? Especially after everything we've talked about so far. But, you'd be surprised how many people out there with diabetes are developing complications simply because they aren't aware of what they can do to prevent these avoidable problems.

Blood Fats

In addition to high blood glucose being a problem for your body, so are certain elevated blood lipid (fat) levels. For example, if your diet is high in fat, especially saturated fat (fat that's solid at room temperature, like butter or shortening), you could eventually develop high cholesterol. That's not a good thing. High cholesterol is known to contribute to the development of plaque in the blood vessels of the heart. This plaque can eventually clog the blood vessels in the heart and cause damage. What does that mean? Well, what happens is piles of this fatty substance called low-density lipoprotein (LDL), also known as the *bad cholesterol*, stick to the inner walls of the blood vessels. The problem is that the LDL plaque may eventually weaken the blood vessel, and if there is enough plaque, it could block blood flow. The plaque in the vessel could even rupture, which would also cause a blockage in blood flow! But that's not all. Plaque can also irritate the blood vessel walls, causing the vessel to spasm (in other words contract), which of course causes further disruption in blood flow. In addition to high cholesterol though, lower levels of high-density lipoprotein (HDL), also know as the *good cholesterol*, can also contribute to this process. You're probably thinking that doesn't make sense! First, high levels of cholesterol are bad then low levels of cholesterol are bad, too! How can that be? Well, we're actually talking about two different types of cholesterol. See, HDL is responsible for carrying the LDL back to the liver so that it can be excreted from the body. But when the levels of HDL are low, there aren't enough of the good guys around to carry the bad guys out!

But that's not all! There's another type of fat that may affect the HDL level called triglycerides. Triglycerides (three fatty acids attached to a glycerol molecule) are the type of fat

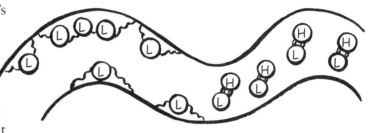

found naturally in food. In addition, the liver also makes triglycerides when excess calories are present. They are transported and stored in the body's fat tissue. The problem with elevated triglycerides is that they are thought to lower HDL levels in some people. What's considered too high of a triglyceride level? Well, for teens with diabetes, anything over 150 mg/dl is too high. So it's important for you to know your numbers and identify your goal. What should your goal be for total cholesterol—LDL and HDL? Well generally speaking for a teen with diabetes the total cholesterol should be less than 170 mg/dl and LDL should be less than 110 mg/dl. The HDL though, needs to be greater than 40 mg/dl for sure, and as you get older, greater that 45 mg/dl for men or 55 mg/dl for women. So you see the goal is to have a lower LDL (bad cholesterol) and a higher level of HDL (good cholesterol). That way we keep the bad guys out and the good guys in!

> If you don't control your blood glucose, you could end up with blood vessel failure and heart complications.
> —Everett

Blood Pressure

Controlling your blood pressure is also something that you should focus on, because hypertension (high blood pressure) can contribute to the development of cardiovascular disease or even kidney complications. Certain individuals are at higher risk for hypertension, such as a person with a strong family history of hypertension or even certain ethnic groups. For example, African Americans are twice as likely to develop hypertension as Caucasians.[4] Not only that, but people with diabetes in general have more incidence of hypertension than those without diabetes. So know your number! What is the magic number? Good question! The American Diabetes Association currently recommends that adults with diabetes maintain a blood pressure of 130/80 mm/hg or less![5] That way you won't have too much force pushing blood through your precious blood vessels. You can do it! Remember a healthy heart is a happy heart!

Smoking

What about smoking? Does smoking affect your blood vessels? You bet it does! The nicotine in cigarettes causes your blood vessels to constrict (become narrower). So what's the big deal about that? Well, think about it, if you have any plaque in your blood vessels (which all of us will have eventually) when you smoke and your blood vessels constrict, you are essentially cutting off the blood supply to your heart! And that's not a good thing! Any time you cut off the blood supply to any cells in your body, the cells can't get oxygen and nutrients needed for survival and will eventually die. So if there's ever a time that you think you might want to smoke, think about what smoking does to your heart.

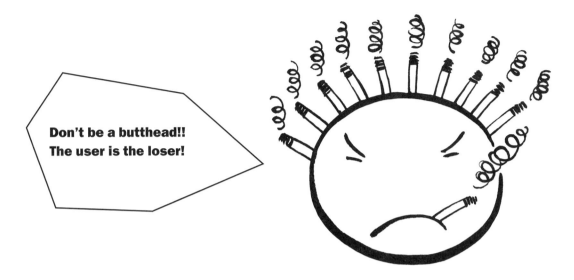

Obesity

Let's not leave out the effect obesity has on your body. Obesity, as you probably already know, has been linked to an increase in cardiovascular (heart and blood vessel) disease. In particular, those people who carry more body weight around their waist are at more risk (especially people with type 2 diabetes). To know where you stand, take a look at your body mass index (BMI). This formula is used to assess body weight in relation to height. It's an important number to know because it correlates pretty closely with body fat. To figure out your BMI you need to take your weight in pounds times 705 then divide by your height in inches squared. Sound confusing—not really. For example, if you're a 180 pound guy and you're 6 feet tall, the formula would look like this: 180 pounds $\times$ 705 = 126,900 divided by 5184 (which is 72 inches squared; or in other words 72 multiplied by itself) = 24.48. A BMI less than 18.5 is considered underweight, 18.5 to 24.9 is healthy, 25.0 to 29.9 is overweight, and 30.0 to 40.0 is considered obese. So, in this example, the 6-foot guy weighing in at 180 pounds ends up with a BMI of 24.48, which is just squeezing in at the healthy weight. But, keep in mind if you are in the overweight category, a weight loss of even 10 to 15 pounds can significantly reduce cardiac risk. Remember, though, it's best to get support and direction from your healthcare professional, because what you don't eat is just as important as what you do eat—do it right!

LET'S DO THE BMI CALCULATION.

6 ft. = 72 in.
180 lbs.

Formula is: **Weight in pounds × 705 ÷ by height in inches squared.**

180 (lbs) × 705 = 126,900

126,900 ÷ 72² (5184) = 24.48 BMI

Activity

That leaves us with activity! Wow, does activity (or lack of activity) ever play a role in the development of the potential complications of diabetes! Just think if a person just gets up and moves, he or she can decrease blood pressure, blood glucose, influence the muscle tone of the heart, and stay in shape! So what kind of activity are we talking about?? Well, it doesn't have to be the *no pain no gain* kinda stuff. Just thirty minutes of any kind of physical activity on most days will give you a huge payoff. And the good news is, it doesn't necessarily have to be all at one time either! So even walking at lunch or to your next class will make a difference in the end. Wouldn't it be cool if instead of seeing people fight over the closest parking spot in front of the mall we saw people fighting over the spot that was the farthest away!! Probably won't happen, but it would be cool! There would probably be a lot less overweight people around, too.

THE COMPLICATIONS OF DIABETES

Okay, we've talked about the major risks associated with the development of diabetes complications. Now let's spend a little time talking specifically about these complications. First let's look at macrovascular complications, in other words those conditions that affect the large blood vessels of the body. Keep focused here—this

Heart Disease

can happen to you! Macrovascular complications can affect the heart, brain, and periphery (arms and legs). To start with we'll focus on the heart and brain because these conditions can be life threatening. As mentioned previously, changes within the blood vessels of the heart and brain occur as a result of uncontrolled diabetes. These changes affect the structure and the function of the blood vessels that feed the heart and brain. And, as you know, anytime there is a disruption of blood flow within an organ (like the heart), that part of the organ will die if no interventions are taken. So what can you do to prevent heart disease or stroke? Well, maintain blood glucose control for one, but there are also other things that can decrease your risk as well. Do you remember the things we talked about before? Things like blood pressure control, watching your cholesterol, and oh yeah, physical activity! Not only that, it's also important for you to continue to get regular physical exams to be sure that you're not developing any problems as you get older. Remember, prevention is the key. And of course, whatever you do—don't smoke! That's like playing Russian roulette—and it's a sure bet that you're not gonna win that one.

Stroke

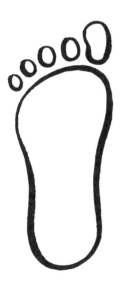

GUIDELINES TO A HEALTHY HEART

- See health care professional regularly.
- Don't smoke.
- Know your numbers—blood glucose level, A1c level (7 percent or less is the goal), blood pressure (130/80 mm/hg or less is the goal for adults), blood lipids (goal for teens: LDL less than 110 mg/dl; total cholesterol less than 170 mg/dl; triglycerides less than 150 mg/dl).
- Keep physically active!! Goal: thirty minutes of activity on most days.
- Maintain a heart healthy weight!
- Eat smart!

Now we'll move on to peripheral vascular disease. What's peripheral vascular disease? Good question! It involves blood vessels in the periphery, like the feet. Peripheral vascular disease isn't usually life threatening, however it can lead to conditions that can be life altering—like infection, gangrene, and even

FOOT CARE GUIDELINES

- Clean, dry, and check your feet every day! What are you checking for??? Good question! Things like blisters or scratches. You know, the regular stuff that happens to feet! If you find something, get it checked out!
- Use a moisturizing lotion on your feet daily (the rest of your body too!). Avoid putting lotion between your toes, because the moisture could promote fungal growth.
- Clip nails straight across and file the corners to the contour of the toe, so they don't dig into the skin of the next toe!
- Never go barefoot—even in the house! Where do you think most injuries occur? In the house!
- Don't cut ingrown toenails yourself.
- Don't ignore foot problems—see your healthcare professional!
- Take your shoes and socks off when you see your healthcare professional, even if you're there for a different reason—take advantage of the opportunity!
- Wear shoes that fit your feet!
- Check the inside of your shoes before you put them on—you never know what you might find!

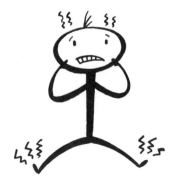

amputations! See, without good blood flow in the periphery there is a risk of poor wound healing because nutrients and oxygen can't get to the injury to do their jobs. Why? Well, remember what we said about plaque that builds up in vessels of the heart and brain? That same thing is happening in other vessels of the body. So, once again, the same prevention strategies make a huge difference! Smoking, for example, is a real problem for people with peripheral vascular disease; so it goes without saying, don't smoke! Remember to take care of your feet, you'll really need them—the average person walks around the world two and half times in his or her lifetime!

Okay, now what's this condition called neuropathy all about? Neuropathy is a condition caused when the body's nerves (which carry impulses throughout the body, similar to an electrical system in a house) are exposed to episodes of high blood glucose over a period of time, coupled with a genetic predisposition and possibly other environmental factors. Most of the time the nervous system involved is the peripheral nervous system, which is made up of the autonomic and sensorimotor nervous systems. You're probably thinking, "What in the heck does that mean?" Well, damage occurs to the nerves, which then interferes with or impairs the way the nerves are supposed to function. It can affect the sensory, motor, or autonomic nerve fibers. Sensorimotor neuropathy usually affects the extremities (arms, hands, legs, or feet). However, if the autonomic nervous system is involved, the person will experience symptoms affecting involuntary functions of the body. This type of neuropathy is referred to as *autonomic neuropathy*. It could potentially affect the gastrointestinal tract (either slow things down or speed things up), the bladder (causing frequent/decreased urination or bladder infections), sexual dysfunction (impotence in males, dryness in females), impaired insulin counterregulation (which can cause unawareness of low blood glucose), or even your blood pressure. Keep in mind neuropathy can even affect both sensorimotor and autonomic nerves at the same time, which is known as diffuse polyneuropathy (multiple nerve involvement). But again, as with everything else that we've discussed so far, the key is *prevention*. Do everything you can to prevent/delay these complications from occurring in the first place. You can do it—you have control!

Sensorimotor neuropathy can literally be a real pain. When neuropathy affects your lower extremities (legs and feet) it can cause the nerves to go a little *haywire*, and that can be painful. But, neuropathy can also interfere with the way the nerve responds to stimuli. For example, typically you would be able to tell if you stepped on a tack, right? Well, if you have neuropathy you may lose what's known as *protective sensation* and you may not be able to feel the pain from the tack in your foot. If you walked around with that tack in your foot for a day or two and it became infected, then you would really have trouble! Now can you see why it's important to check your feet every day? If you have neuropathy that affects your feet, you really need to be extra careful.

Okay, that brings us to kidney disease, a.k.a. diabetic nephropathy. Approximately 40 to 50 percent of people who have had type 1 diabetes for more than twenty years develop some form of nephropathy.[6] But, if after twenty-five or thirty years of having diabetes that person still hasn't developed nephropathy, then he or she is less likely to develop it in the future. So let's focus on that!!!

First let's talk about what happens with diabetic nephropathy. You know that everybody has two kidneys. The kidneys are responsible for filtering waste from the body's blood (forming urine), maintaining blood volume, regulating blood pressure, maintaining acid-base balance, making the hormone erythropoietin (which in turn stimulates red blood cell formation), and finally processes vitamin D (which is needed to absorb calcium). Okay, after saying all that, let's focus on what can happen to the kidneys when a person has diabetes—diabetic nephropathy.

There are several factors that may be involved in the development of diabetic nephropathy. As with the other complications associated with diabetes, though, it is likely that high blood glucose plays a part. For example, when the kidneys are exposed to periods of high blood glucose over time, changes start to occur within the structure of the kidneys. These changes occur in the nephron (special cells in the kidney) and involve the glomerulus (tiny blood vessels), which are responsible for blood filtration. Changes in the structure of the blood vessels of the kidney tend to occur more frequently in people with type 1 diabetes. In addition, rates of nephropathy are three to six times higher for African Americans, Hispanics, and Native Americans, and there is also an increase incidence of nephropathy in people over the age of sixty.[7]

STAGES OF DIABETIC NEPHROPATHY

- Stage I—kidneys are working harder to filter blood. Glucose control can reverse this stage.
- Stage II—changes occurring in the kidney. Glucose control can still reverse this stage.
- Stage III—both structural and functional changes in the kidney lead to abnormal filtration, so microalbumin (tiny protein particles) are seen in urine with a special test. There are usually no symptoms yet.
- Stage IV—abnormal filtration gets worse. Now protein is easily found in the urine. High blood pressure and nephrotic syndrome (weight gain, swelling of the feet, and congestive heart failure) develop.
- Stage V—known as end-stage renal disease. Kidneys can no longer filter the blood properly so the person must receive kidney dialysis (artificial blood filtering process) or a kidney transplant to survive.

The risk factors for developing diabetic nephropathy include poor blood glucose control, duration of diabetes, high blood pressure (further damages the blood vessels), genetic predisposition, and smoking (not a surprise). Three of the five major risk factors are modifiable, so you can do something to prevent or delay the onset of diabetic nephropathy! Okay, what can you do? Make sure you are doing all you can to reach your blood glucose goals. Also, see your healthcare professional regularly. This is especially important because there is a test that can be done to identify early kidney disease, when it is still reversible. That's right, early diabetic nephropathy can be reversed! For example, sometimes medication is prescribed to prevent or delay the progression of diabetic nephropathy. In addition, if the person has hypertension, early, aggressive treatment of the high blood pressure can also prevent progression, especially early in the disease. Still in others, dietary restriction of protein may be prescribed to help prevent or delay the progression of the disease. If dietary restriction is recommended by your healthcare professional, make sure you see a dietitian who has experience in kidney disease. This type of meal plan requires special attention to detail, so you will benefit from a dietitian who has worked with people with kidney disease previously. Also, try to prevent urinary tract infections so as to prevent further injury to the kidneys. And remember—don't smoke!!

TIPS TO PREVENT URINARY TRACT INFECTIONS

- Females should wipe from front to back after urinating to prevent contaminating the urethra from the rectum.
- Drinking cranberry juice may help to acidify the urine and has shown to decrease the incidence of urinary tract infections in susceptible individuals.
- Know the signs and symptoms of a urinary tract infection, like burning when urinating or frequent urination.
- See your healthcare professional if you develop any symptoms—don't wait!

Now all we have left to talk about is diabetic eye disease. The most prevalent diabetic eye disease is diabetic retinopathy, which can and does occur in teens. This disease occurs when the tiny blood vessels that feed the retina (nerves in the back of the eye where focusing occurs) are damaged, allowing blood to leak out of the vessels into the retina. As with nephropathy, retinopathy is categorized into stages that include nonproliferative (nonspreading) and proliferative (spreading) retinopathy.

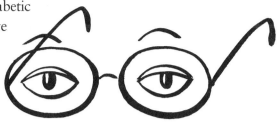

Let's start with proliferative retinopathy, because this is the type of retinopathy that causes more problems. When retinopathy is allowed to progress, new blood vessels develop on the surface of the retina to make up for damaged vessels. Unfortunately, these vessels are very fragile and break easily, causing hemorrhages and even retinal detachment in some cases. As a result, there is a range of visual changes and/or loss of vision that can occur depending on the degree and location of the new growth and subsequent hemorrhages.

Nonproliferative retinopathy, on the other hand, can range from mild to severe, but it does not involve the development of

OTHER EYE COMPLICATIONS ASSOCIATED WITH DIABETES

- ◎ Cataracts (lens of the eye becomes opaque) occur more frequently and at a younger age in people with diabetes.
- ◎ Open-angled glaucoma (increased pressure in the eye, which impairs vision and may slowly cause eye damage and vision loss).
- ◎ Eye palsies (nerves of the eye are affected, causing impairment of the muscle around the eye—temporary).
- ◎ Blurred vision due to uncontrolled blood glucose (resolves with return of blood glucose control).
- ◎ Visual changes such as dim vision, flashing lights, or double vision can occur during low blood glucose.

new blood vessels. The classic signs of nonproliferative retinopathy include the development of pouches in weak blood vessel walls. There may also be accumulation of fat particles and fluid that leaks through the walls of the blood vessels onto the retina. In the mild form of nonproliferative retinopathy, vision is usually not affected. If the disease progresses, more damage occurs, which can lead to the development of proliferative retinopathy.

It's no surprise that prevention is the key. A dilated eye exam by a trained optometrist or ophthalmologist to examine the retina is worth its weight in gold! The exam is simple; it just involves putting drops in the eyes that cause the pupils to become larger so the physician can look at the retina with a special light. This is the only time a healthcare professional can look at the vessels in your body without cutting you open! But remember, this exam can only be performed when your eyes have been dilated. Once again, not enough can be said for the benefits of blood glucose, blood pressure, and blood lipid control. And of course, let's just say it one more time—don't smoke!

Once retinopathy develops though, there are various treatment options available. For example, in the case of mild nonproliferative retinopathy the treatment includes observation. There are also various tests/procedures that may be performed to document the stage and progression of the disease. In addition, in cases where blood vessels are leaking and vision is in jeopardy a procedure may be recommended to seal the leaking blood vessels. People who have proliferative retinopathy may receive laser treatments to reduce severe vision loss or if the retinopathy includes the vitreous (jellylike mass that fills the eye), the healthcare practitioner may recommend surgical removal of the vitreous. In this case the vitreous will then be replaced with a clear solution.

So you can see there are multiple treatments available to help a person who has retinopathy. It's wonderful that we have such successful treatments available at our fingertips; now we just have to get people in for screening. Current statistics affirm that more than 90 percent of vision loss could be prevented with proper treatment. Don't be another statistic!

NOTES

1. The DCCT Research Group, "The Effect of Intensive Treatment of Diabetes on the Development and Progression of Long-Term Complications in Insulin-Dependent Diabetes Mellitus," *New England Journal of Medicine* 329, (1993): 977–86.

2. National Diabetes Information Clearinghouse, "What Is the DCCT?" available at www.niddk.nih.gov/health/diabetes/pubs/dcct1/dcct.htm (January 10, 2003).

3. Martha M. Funnell, Cheryl Hunt, Karmeen Kulkarni, Richard R. Rubin, and Peggy C. Yarborough, *A Core Curriculum for Diabetes Education* (Chicago: American Association of Diabetes Educators, 1998), 661.

4. Funnell et al., *A Core Curriculum for Diabetes Education*, 662.

5. American Diabetes Association, "Treatment of Hypertension in Adults with Diabetes," *Diabetes Care* 25, Supplement 1 (January 2002): S71.

6. Marion J. Franz, Karmeen Kulkarni, William H. Polonsky, Peggy Yarborough, and Virginia Zamudio, *A Core Curriculum for Diabetes Education: Diabetes Management Therapies* (Chicago: American Association of Diabetes Educators, 2001), 157.

7. Franz et al., *A Core Curriculum for Diabetes Education*, 153.

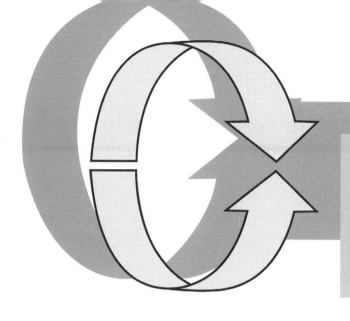

You've probably thought to yourself at one point or another, "Can I do this on my own?" Well, there's no need to worry, because you don't have to! You can use the diabetes healthcare team! Having diabetes can be a real pain! It requires a lot of planning, organization, and responsibility. It's a daunting task for anyone. But remember, you don't have to do all the planning, organization, and detective work on your own. There is a wealth of resources available at your fingertips. It's just a matter of hooking up with the right people. Healthcare professionals are like a good pair of shoes; you just have to find a pair that fits well on you! But, in order to find those special people, you're gonna have to know yourself as well. Let's talk about that for a minute.

WHAT'S YOUR TYPE?

Are you the type of person that likes to be totally *independent*? Do you always want things to be perfect? Are you moral, honest, and truthful, but tend to be critical of yourself and maybe even others? Are all those little details in life really important to you? Maybe you're the person everyone else looks to for guidance? Pretty hard to ask for help when you're the one that's usually giving it out isn't it? Well, that's understandable. But remember, you are not alone on this earth and even though this sounds harsh, no one is perfect (in fact, it's not a perfect world). Remember one thing, we're all human. Your drive for perfection and attention to detail will help you to be organized in your diabetes management and it will help you stay on course. But, don't expect perfection 100 percent of the time in your diabetes control; set realistic goals. Step out of the box long enough to reach out for support from those around you!

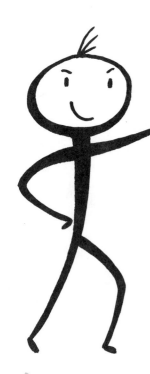

Maybe you're the *quiet* type. You know, the one who likes to sit in the background and watch what's going on around you—just taking it all in. Do you appreciate wisdom, knowledge, and education? Are you always trying to understand the world; always looking at how things work? Maybe you're the one people refer to as the sensible one because you tend to communicate clearly and succinctly, yet you're comfortable being alone as well. If so, just be careful not to remove yourself too much from those who are there to support you. If you do, you may run the risk of being in a perpetual state of planning. That's a problem, because you'll end up being distracted from focusing, deciding, and actually doing!

Perhaps you're the *take-charge* type. Do you tend to be very direct and maybe even frank with people? Are you always searching for the truth or justice in situations? Do you feel like you're constantly in a battle as you make your way through life? Or do you sometimes even take this search for justice to extremes? Do people say that you're really energetic and captivating? You will benefit most by trying to focus your energy into strategies that will give you the biggest payoff in the end. Remember, there has been a lot of effort put into research that has proven aggressive diabetes management yields positive outcomes. This truth has already

WHAT'S A NATIONAL YOUTH ADVOCATE?

- A youth advocate serves as a spokesperson for the American Diabetes Association and travels all over the United States.
- He or she will meet with policymakers to promote increased funding for diabetes research and talk to a lot of people along the way!
- So if you're passionate about finding a cure for diabetes and you're not afraid to talk about it, call the American Diabetes Association!

1-800-DIABETES

been proven. So, you can capitalize on the energy that's already been invested in this research and apply these practices to your everyday life, with a little support from the healthcare team.

Or maybe you're a *follow-the-crowd* type and you're really just along for the ride. Do you believe that you are at peace, union, and oneness with your world? Do you find yourself thinking about life in general or about your diabetes as "what's the big deal, it doesn't matter, we're not here that long anyway"? Or maybe you find yourself settling for the status quo (same old, same old). Well, the truth of the matter is we (human beings) won't live forever, and in the scope of things, we are really not here that long. And because we're not, you need to make the most of what you have available to you today! See, it really is a big deal because you have tools available to you that will make your life easier. Take advantage of life! Remember, you are in control!

Maybe you're not any of those other types. Maybe you're the type that likes to *beat your own drum*! You know, the type that loves to experience life and create your own fun and happiness. Maybe you always have a new idea and have the

123

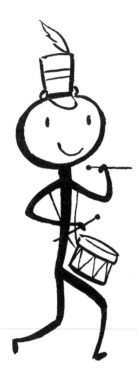

desire and ability to move quickly on those ideas. Do you like your life to be fast-paced? Or, do you tend to really blossom when you have a lot of variety or external stimulation in your life? Have you ever thought that maybe this fast pace is related to the anxiety you have about life? See, sometimes people like to distract themselves and others so that they don't have to deal with what they are really thinking or feeling. Don't let this be you. This is not psychological mumbo jumbo; it's just that sometimes people who are dancing through life really fast are actually trying to run away from something. Don't feel like you have to run, especially if there are issues related to your diabetes that are making you *dance* fast. Stop and hook-up with one of the healthcare team members. Really, this is not something you have to dance through alone.

HEALTH CARE TEAM

Okay, so who is a part of this healthcare team we've been talking about? Well to begin with, the primary care physician. This is the person that you can see for everyday kinda stuff: like a bad cough, sore throat, or even a broken arm. There are even primary care physicians out there that have a lot of experience working with people with diabetes. If you have the kind of provider that can take care of all that stuff and help you manage your diabetes as well, that's great. If you don't have that kind of provider, then ask to see an endocrinologist who can help you manage your diabetes.

What's an endocrinologist? Good question! An endocrinologist is a physician who specializes in diabetes management, as well as other endocrine disorders. This person not only helps you manage your diabetes, but can also make sure you're not developing any complications from the disease.

WHAT SHOULD I EXPECT WHEN I GO TO SEE THE ENDOCRINOLOGIST?

First, the endocrinologist will ask you questions about your medical history and risk factors. For example, he or she will talk to you about your eating patterns, maybe even look at your weight and growth history. The endocrinologist may also ask if you smoke, drink alcohol, or if you're sexually active. During this time, it's important to tell the endocrinologist about your health beliefs. Like maybe you're really upset about having diabetes and you have things on your mind that are worrying you. Don't be afraid to tell your physician and ask questions—remember there's no such thing as a stupid question!

If you've already had diabetes for some time, but you are going to the endocrinologist for the first time, the physician may ask you about your previous treatment. For example the physician may ask you questions like "What types of medications/insulin do you take?" "What is your meal plan?" "What's your typical exercise routine?" What's your A1c?" He or she will probably also ask for your blood glucose monitoring results and what changes you made in your plan based on those results.

Then he or she will do a comprehensive physical assessment. You know, the regular kind of checkup you're used to getting from your primary care physician. For example, he or she will look at your blood pressure, height, weight, listen to your heart, look in your mouth, throat, and eyes, feel your abdomen, and look at your feet. You can also expect blood work to be done. For example, your physician will likely order an A1c level, fasting lipid (blood fat) profile, thyroid stimulating hormone (there is an increase in thyroid disease in people who already have autoimmune disorders like type 1 diabetes), and maybe a serum creatinine to check kidney function. The physician is also likely to order a urinalysis for ketones, protein, and sediment and a test for microalbuminuria if you've had diabetes for five years or more.

The endocrinologist may also refer you to a specialist, based on the results of his or her findings. So for example, if you were diagnosed with diabetes within the past three to five years or if you've had diabetes for longer than that, but haven't had a dilated eye exam in the past year, then a referral for an eye exam by an ophthalmologist or optometrist who is knowledgeable and experienced in diagnosing diabetic retinopathy is indicated. If you have a problem with your feet that the endocrinologist can't help you with, then a referral to a foot specialist is indicated. Or let's say you haven't had any diabetes education before, or it's been a couple of years since you last had diabetes education, then a referral to a certified diabetes educator is indicated. Certainly, if you've never seen a dietitian about your individualized meal plan or if it's been a while (over a year) since you've reviewed your meal plan, then a referral to a dietitian is indicated.

WHAT SHOULD I EXPECT WHEN I GO TO SEE THE CERTIFIED DIABETES EDUCATOR (CDE) AND REGISTERED DIETITIAN (RD)?

A certified diabetes educator specializes in educating the person with diabetes and his or her significant others on diabetes and its management. This person can be a registered nurse, registered dietitian, social worker, pharmacist, exercise physiologist, or physician who has been certified through national credentialing to provide comprehensive diabetes management education. As you can see, the certified diabetes educator comes to the table with a wealth of knowledge and experience helping people, like you, with their diabetes.

So, what can you expect when you see the certified diabetes educator? Well, the CDE will ask you questions regarding your past medical history and risk factors, take your blood pressure, weight, and height, and take a look at recent blood work results from your primary care physician or endocrinologist. The CDE will also assess your current knowledge level regarding diabetes and its management to determine what you *need* help with and to determine what you *want* help with. He or she may also ask you questions regarding your health beliefs, health practices, and current treatment plan, if you have one.

Then you and the CDE will come up with a plan. This plan will identify the areas that you need assistance with regarding diabetes management. Afterward, the CDE will provide you with information to help you manage your diabetes, based on the plan. There will be opportunities for you to ask questions

IN THE SPOTLIGHT
CYNTHIA FRITCHIE, RN, MS, CDE

I was diagnosed with type 1 at age 2 (1965)! My sister who is one year younger than I was born with downs syndrome and a heart defect. My parents were told she would not live a year. (This will all come together.) In Nov. of 1965, my parents took a much-needed trip to Egypt. This was during the age when flights only went 1–2 times/week. My aunt was staying with me, my sister, and my newborn brother. I started showing the classic symptoms of diabetes—standing by the sink and begging for water—only leaving to pee and return to the sink! My aunt took me to the hospital where they discovered the diabetes. She sent a telegram to Egypt—"daughter very sick, come home at once." My parents thought the telegram was about my little sister and went to the American embassy to help them get home faster. By the time they arrived in Chicago, 2 days later, they were so relieved to find out it was me with diabetes and not Vicky dying from her heart condition!

I started out as an actress with a bachelors degree in fine arts in theater from New York University, but soon realized I could not earn a living doing that. In the early 1990s I went to Rush University in Chicago for my bachelors and masters in nursing. I became a certified diabetes educator in 1994 and never looked back.

Currently, I am the project manager for a National Institutes of Health–funded study at the University of Illinois at Chicago College of Nursing. The study is called "Cardiovascular Risks in Adolescents with Diabetes." We are studying exercise capacity testing, lipid profiles, nutrition, and something called Heart Rate Variability, which looks at changes in the heart's nervous system. We are comparing kids with type 1 to kids with type 2 diabetes.

I have 2 sons (George and Henry) who were born early. They're both healthy now at ages 5 and 7. Last year, my husband Paul and I traveled to China to adopt a little girl: Anne Li Xiang. She is a clown from the word go and keeps us running. An absolute terror, my mother nicknamed her "typhoon Annie." She is a joy, but I can't wait until the terrible 2s are behind us!

We are a traveling family and I have taken my insulin and supplies all around the world. My pump has been plunged into the Aegean, Mediterranean, Atlantic, and Pacific oceans and has kept me level through many time zones, climates, and exotic food experiences. I hope to stay active in diabetes care and research all my life, or until a Broadway director calls!

and even practice what you've learned. So, take advantage of the opportunity! And don't think that once you're done with the instruction you won't be able to rely on this person to help you with issues that come up through your life regarding your diabetes management. That's what they're there for, to help you with your diabetes management. So as you can see, the CDE isn't someone that you see just once and then you're out of there! He or she is really someone who can help you work on the areas that you may have difficulty with in your diabetes management throughout your lifetime.

During the consultation, the CDE will ask you to come up with a couple of goals that you would like to work on. For example, perhaps you want to learn about *hypoglycemia unawareness* because you've had a couple of low blood glucose experiences while driving that you didn't recognize. As a result of that experience, maybe you decide your goal will be to check your blood glucose without fail before driving your car for the next month. Or, maybe you were just recently diagnosed with diabetes and you want to learn about the meal plan. And, let's say the CDE recommends that you make a couple of nutrition changes. For example, maybe instead of drinking regular soda with breakfast, lunch, and dinner (yuk!), you decide that your goal is to only drink ½ cup of regular soda with lunch two or three days out of the week for the next month, or maybe you want to give up regular soda altogether.

What about the registered dietitian? Well, as we discussed previously, the registered dietitian can also be a CDE who specializes in nutrition management for people with diabetes. This person can really help you make good nutrition choices. The registered dietitian will focus on that part of your diabetes management that involves what you eat! Everyone must eat to survive, right? Yes, but what you eat can make a huge difference in how healthy you are. The dietitian's job is to help you understand how the food you eat

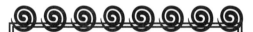

Monday—for breakfast I had 2 cups of cereal with ½ cup of milk, a banana, and 1 slice of toast with 1 tsp. of jelly. Lunch I skipped because I was late for my dance class. So, I had a snack around 2:00 P.M.—small bag of chips and carton of chocolate milk. Then I was really hungry at dinner (around 6:30 P.M.). Had a couple handfuls of cheese puffs while I was waiting for dinner. Then I had two pieces of chicken, 1 cup of mashed potatoes and gravy, about ½ cup of beans and a slice of bread with margarine. And a 6 oz. glass of milk. I didn't have my snack before bed (still full and my blood glucose was high).

IN THE SPOTLIGHT
ROBIN ANN WILLIAMS, MA, RD, CDE

When were you diagnosed with type 1?
1974—I was 26 years old

Where did you get your degree?
Bachelors of science—University of California–Davis,
master in arts—San Jose State University

Where do you practice now?
Northern Michigan in a mostly rural setting

I was married for 3 years before I was diagnosed with diabetes.
My husband and I have two boys, one born in 1978 (before
there were blood glucose monitors—he was 11 lbs, 5 oz) and
one born 1980 (he was 8 lbs 3 oz with no complications—I had a
blood glucose monitor for this one!)

I did diabetes education in private practice in California for
about 10 years. Then I moved around in the Midwest for a while,
but finally settled in Michigan. We also have two dogs.

For fun I like to knit, white water and wilderness canoe. I'm
also a high adventure leader in the Boy Scouts of America.

affects your diabetes management, your health status, and even
your energy level! So, you can see that there is some truth to
that old saying, "You are what you eat!"

It's best if you can come to the dietitian with a log of what
you typically eat in a day; including the snacks and little treats
here and there. Try to be as truthful and complete as you can; it
will only help you out in the long run. And don't be afraid to
tell the dietitian that you can't live without cookies or French
fries. He or she will be able to work your favorites into your
meal plan without a problem. Now, that doesn't mean you can
feel free to eat junk 24/7, nobody should! But, what it does
mean is that it's possible to work anything you want into your
meal plan; it's all about when you eat it (like what your blood
glucose level is when you decide to have a couple of cookies)
and the amount that you eat (you need to learn about
carbohydrates and what a real serving size is—and no, a pound
of French fries is not one serving!).

WHAT SHOULD I EXPECT WHEN I GO TO SEE THE OPHTHALMOLOGIST OR OPTOMETRIST?

The ophthalmologist or optometrist will do a compete evaluation, including a dilated eye exam. To begin, the specialist will probably check your visual acuity (how well you are able to see) by asking you to read letters on a wall chart from varying distances. You know the routine, "Please cover your left eye and read the first line." After that he or she may do a test to check for glaucoma (a condition that can lead to blindness if there is damage to the optic nerve), which involves checking the pressure in your eyes. Some glaucoma tests involve touching a tonometer to your eye (instrument that measures pressure in your eye). This type of test requires eye drops that numb the eye before the test. Another technique used to check for glaucoma uses the air puff method, which doesn't require the eye numbing drops first. It just depends on which method your practitioner prefers. After the glaucoma test, eye drops that dilate your pupils will be used so that the physician can see the retina in

---

OPHTHALMOLOGIST/OPTOMETRIST, WHAT'S THE DIFFERENCE?

- An ophthalmologist is a medical doctor who diagnoses, treats, and studies diseases of the eye.
- An optometrist is specifically trained and skilled in examining the eyes, testing visual acuity, and prescribing corrective lenses.
- Both can diagnose retinopathy and other conditions of the eye, but treatment may need to be referred to an ophthalmologist.

E

F P

L P E D

P E C F D

E D F C Z P

D E F P O T E C

the back of your eyes using an ophthalmoscope. This instrument allows the physician to check for eye disease such as retinopathy (damage to the retina) or cataracts (cloudy lens). That's it!

Make sure you bring a pair of sunglasses with you so that you won't have trouble seeing when you're done. It takes a couple of hours for your pupils to return to the normal size after the exam; during that time it will be difficult to read things close up. You shouldn't have trouble driving, although it may be a good idea to bring someone with you to drive just in case.

WHAT SHOULD I EXPECT WHEN I GO TO SEE THE NEPHROLOGIST?

The nephrologist is a physician who specializes in treating diseases of the kidney. Just like when you saw the endocrinologist, the nephrologist will do a medical history and physical examination that will likely be very similar to what you have experienced with the endocrinologist. He or she will also probably order special tests to determine if you have kidney disease or, if you know you have kidney disease, to determine the degree of kidney disease you already have. These tests may include blood work such as blood urea nitrogen (BUN) and creatinine to determine kidney function. The specialist will also order a urinalysis (urine test) to check for large or small amounts of protein. A 24-hour urine for microalbuminuria and 24-hour urine for creatinine clearance (two separate tests) may also be ordered to determine early kidney disease and current kidney function. For a 24-hour urine test, you simply need to collect all of your urine for a 24-hour period of time, keep it cold while you're collecting it, then return the specimen to the clinic or laboratory. The 24-hour urine for microalbuminuria is a very sensitive test that will be able to pick up very early kidney disease, when it can still be reversed! In some cases the specialist may also order an ultrasound of the kidneys to see if there are any physical abnormalities with the size and/or shape of the kidneys, or to determine if a tumor is present.

WHAT SHOULD I EXPECT WHEN I GO TO SEE THE DENTIST?

Let's hope that by now you've had the experience of seeing a dentist and dental hygienist for a dental evaluation and cleaning. The routine for a diabetes dental evaluation is no different from what you've experienced in the past. Dental x-rays will probably be taken to see if any tooth decay is present, then the hygienist will evaluate and clean your teeth. After the hygienist is finished, the dentist will perform a comprehensive dental evaluation to determine if there are any oral tissue or tooth abnormalities present. The dentist may ask you questions regarding your oral health as part of this comprehensive dental evaluation, too. For example, he or she may ask if your gums ever bleed, feel swollen or tender, or if any of your teeth are loose. He or she may also ask if you have a problem with persistent bad breath or if you smoke.

It's important for you to see a dentist every six months because of the increased risk for periodontal disease (inflammation of the supporting structures of the teeth) in people with diabetes, such as gingivitis (inflammation of the gums). Again, prevention is the key! See your dentist regularly, brush, floss, and control those blood glucose levels!

WHAT SHOULD I EXPECT WHEN I GO TO SEE THE CARDIOLOGIST?

The cardiologist is a physician who specializes in diagnosing and treating heart disease. Once again, this specialist will likely ask you questions regarding your medical history and risk factors and will perform a comprehensive physical assessment, similar to the endocrinologist. The purpose of this referral is to determine what, if any, changes are occurring in your cardiovascular system that may put you at risk for complications.

You can expect the specialist to order blood work (see a pattern here?) if you haven't had recent blood work completed.

For example, he or she may request a lipid panel to evaluate the blood fats (remember elevated total cholesterol, LDL, triglycerides, and low HDL put you at risk for cardiovascular disease). Perhaps the specialist will order liver enzymes, BUN, and creatinine to determine if there are any underlying conditions of the liver or kidneys that may complicate your care, and maybe a complete blood count to determine if there are any current infections, anemia (condition in which the number of blood cells, blood cell volume, or hemoglobin is less than normal), or other conditions currently affecting your health status. The cardiologist may also order an electrocardiogram (EKG), which records the heart's electrical currents, a stress test (to see how the heart responds before, during, and after stress), or even an echocardiogram (a type of ultrasound used to identify abnormalities in the heart's structure and function).

WHAT SHOULD I EXPECT WHEN I GO TO SEE THE NEUROLOGIST?

A neurologist is a specialist in the diagnosis and treatment of nervous system disease. This is the person you would be referred to if you were having symptoms of neuropathy, such as a burning sensation in your hands or feet, or problems with urination, digestion, or even dizziness. The neurologist will determine where the nerve damage is and hopefully help to alleviate or at least help you live with the problem through treatment.

He or she will determine whether you have diabetic neuropathy, based on the results of the physical examination and medical history, which is similar to what you've already experienced with your primary care physician. The neurologist will ask you questions about your symptoms such as the type of symptoms, how long you've had the symptoms, and if anything makes the symptoms better or worse. During the physical exam, he or she may check your response to sensation by using a Semmes-Weinstein 5.07 monofilament. You're probably thinking, "What in the heck is that?" Well, it's really just a piece of nylon fiber that the physician will touch to the end of your toe or bottom of your foot to see if you can feel it or not. Don't worry it doesn't hurt; it's about the same type of material as fishing line. He or she may also check to see if you can feel a change in temperature by putting something cool on your foot. In addition, there's an instrument called a tuning fork (no, it's not a real fork!) that can be used to check if you have any loss in vibration sensation. Expect the physician to check your muscle strength, your reflexes, and your blood pressure, and pulse as you move to different positions (lying down, then sitting and standing). The neurologist will also look at your feet to see if there are any changes in the structure, in the appearance of the skin, or in the blood supply (can be done by looking at and touching the foot). Expect to have blood work done because sometimes the cause for the symptoms is related to something other than diabetes. So, for example the physician may order a complete blood count, electrolyte levels (things like potassium, calcium, sodium), thyroid function tests, or a sedimentation rate to see if there is an inflammatory condition of the blood vessels causing the symptoms. He or she may even order tests for B_{12}, folic acid, and other vitamin and mineral deficiencies. In addition, if you have risk factors for sexually transmitted diseases, like syphilis or HIV, the neurologist may order these blood tests as well.

In some circumstances, an electromyography (EMG) and nerve conduction study may be used to see if there is any nerve or muscle damage. This test looks at how well the nerves and muscles are working by putting little electrodes on or in the skin and muscle of the affected area. The function of the nerve and muscle are checked by having you tense and relax the muscle in the area and by applying a small electrical pulse to the affected nerve. Sounds like something from a Frankenstein movie doesn't it? Don't worry it's not!

There is really no way to monitor for autonomic neuropathy, so it's important to tell the physician if you ever have problems with digestion, urination, sweating, dizziness, or things like that. If you have problems with urination for example, the physician may order a urinalysis and culture to check for infection, and/or an ultrasound or x-ray of the bladder or urinary system to find out why you're having the symptoms.

Just remember, the best treatment for any complication of diabetes is prevention. Pay attention to what your body is telling you! Above all, enlist the help of healthcare professionals who have a lot of experience in diabetes management, as well as treatment of complications of diabetes. There's no reason to depend on hindsight where diabetes complications are concerned—medical science has the knowledge and tools; it's your job to hook into them!

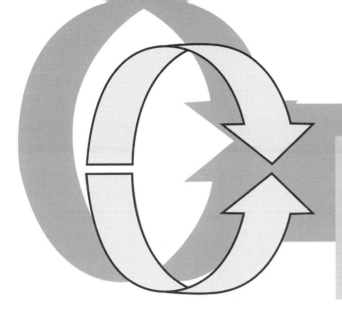

Chapter 14
Peers, Beers, and Tears

You know what it's like. You're at a party when a friend comes up to you and says, "Hey bud, gotcha a beer." So, what's your response? "No thanks" and then you quickly come up with some excuse why you're not drinking, or maybe you say "Thanks man" and quickly guzzle the beer down, or maybe you thank your friend, take the beer, but just hold on to it for the rest of the night. Any of these scenarios sound familiar? If not, have you thought about what you would do in this situation? Well, the best way to deal with a situation like this one is to have a plan. Yeah, a

plan. What that means is, you better think about it and you better come up with a solution that works for you.

To begin, let's talk about whether it's okay for you to drink alcohol. First of all you know that in most states the legal drinking age is twenty-one. Okay, so if you're not twenty-one (really) then legally you can't drink. Okay, having said that now let's look at what's really happening with teens

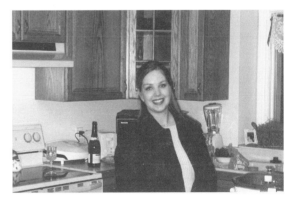

in the United States. Are they drinking? Yes. So, what should *you* do? Glad you asked!!

PEERS AND BEERS

Chances are pretty good that eventually you'll be faced with this dilemma, "To drink or not to drink?" That is the question!

Keeping face around your friends is important, of course! But, so is having all the facts and making an informed decision. So let's look at the facts. Alcohol affects everyone differently. It's a well-known fact that men and women experience different physiological effects of alcohol. For example, women become intoxicated quicker. That's because women have less overall water content in their bodies (so there's less fluid to dilute the alcohol). In addition, an enzyme called *alcohol dehydrogenase* is less active in women.[1] The purpose of this enzyme (found in the stomach) is to break down alcohol so that it can be excreted from the body.

Okay, what effect does alcohol have on diabetes? Well, alcohol has an equal response on men and women where diabetes is concerned. See, when you drink alcohol your liver is really busy trying to get rid of the toxins (alcohol) so it isn't able to respond physically to the body's needs the way it should. For example, if your blood glucose level starts to drop, the body's normal response is to stimulate the liver, by way of the autonomic nervous system. Your liver then releases little blurbs of stored glucose in response to the emergency. In this circumstance, though, the liver is already busy, so it can't respond the way it should. To make matters worse, your brain, which usually tries to tell you that your blood glucose level is dropping (by making you feel dizzy, unsteady, or even sweaty), can't get the message across either, because the alcohol masks the symptoms! So you are literally up a creek without a paddle!

So what can you do? Well, remember you can just say no, but if you choose to drink, you must drink responsibly. What does that mean? Well, don't drink and drive (of course) and don't drink too much! A good rule of thumb to follow is the one-drink limit. And be smart; don't drink without eating! This is not the time to risk having a low blood glucose level. You should also check your blood glucose level frequently and have something to eat before you go to bed as well. Another important thing to remember is not to drink by yourself. You really need to have someone with you in the event you begin to have symptoms of low blood glucose but don't recognize it.

You may be wondering what you can do if you really don't want to drink, but your friends continue to pressure you. Well, sometimes you really need to stand up for what you believe in. But, sometimes the time just isn't right. If that's the case, try pretending. Yep, pretend by keeping your glass half full all night, no one will notice that you're not actually drinking out of the glass. It looks like you're drinking because the glass is only half full! See, it's really true, where there's a will there's a way. Remember, everyone needs an out now and then. Go with what works for you and don't worry about it! Hey, here's an even better idea—volunteer to be the designated driver! Remember—drinking and driving is stupid for anyone.

Yep! Smoking is just like a smokin' gun. Nope, I'm not gonna cut any slack on this one. Smoking will accelerate the complications of diabetes and even create a few more of its own. Surely you've heard of emphysema, chronic obstructive pulmonary disease, or the big "C" cancer. But did you know that smoking, when you have diabetes, is especially detrimental? It's really like playing Russian roulette. Yeah, it's true. See, smoking accelerates the microvascular and macrovascular complications of diabetes. So, it's not like, "Well maybe I won't get those complications," it's really like, "When will I get those complications?" Not only that, but there's also an increased risk of premature death, too.

So where does that leave you? Well, if you don't smoke, then whatever you do don't start! If your friends are smoking, get them to stop—friends listen to friends. Ya know, you could be saving their lives! This is certainly a battle that's worth fighting. It won't be easy, that's for sure—but it's worth it.

What if you are already smoking? Stop! Do whatever it takes, but do it now! Your life depends on it. Go see your healthcare professional today. There are lots of different things out there to help you get through the addiction (yeah, it's definitely an addiction). For example, nicotine

Smoking is directly responsible for 87 percent of lung cancer.

Smoking accounts for 440,000 deaths each year!

Smoking is the leading avoidable cause of death in the United States.[2]

Approximately 4.5 million U.S. teens smoke; 22.4 percent of high school seniors smoke daily. Ninety percent of smokers begin smoking before the age of twenty-one.

Smoking costs the U.S. $150 billion a year in healthcare costs and lost productivity.

Cigarettes contain at least forty-three distinct cancer-causing chemicals.[3]

replacement therapy (patches) has been effective in helping people quit smoking. But, what really helps is getting some behavioral counseling, too. Sounds freaky, right? Well it's not, really! That just means you go to someone who helps you figure out ways to curb the cravings and, in the end, really increases your chances of being successful! Remember one thing if you're a smoker—never quit quitting! If you try something and it just doesn't work, then try something else, until it does work.

Smoking makes complications happen faster. It will kill you. —Nicole

TIPS TO HELP YOU QUIT

Here is a list of things to help you kick the habit:

- Set a date for quitting and stick to it!! Maybe you can even get one of your friends who smokes to quit with you—two heads are better than one!

- Try to figure out what circumstances make you want to smoke more and address them—maybe it's stress, or boredom, or when you're hungry?

- Only allow yourself to smoke when you're outside, not in the car, not when you're watching TV, not when you're talking on the phone.

- Smoke only half of the cigarette and throw the remainder away.

- Cut back in the number of cigarettes you smoke in a day—let's say fifteen instead of twenty. Then the next week make it ten instead of fifteen and so on.

- Don't bum cigarettes from others!

- For goodness sake throw away all of your cigarettes and get rid of anything that reminds you of smoking—like your lighter perhaps!!

- Stay focused and stay busy!

- Always have other things available to curb your craving for a cigarette—maybe some sugar-free gum?

- Reward yourself at the end of the day for not smoking, or maybe you could save the money you're not spending on cigarettes and buy yourself something at the end of the month!

- Tell your friends that you've quit smoking. You'll need your friends to support you.

SEX, STDS, PREGNANCY, AND YOU

What does "STD" mean? It stands for sexually transmitted disease. There are a lot of them out there and they're sneaky. You really need to be smart about this kind of stuff. So listen up!!

Most sexually transmitted diseases are types of infections that are spread from person to person. A disease is considered sexually transmitted when it is passed from person to person through intimate sexual contact. STDs include things like chlamydia, herpes, gonorrhea, syphilis, HIV, yes even HIV. What's really important to remember is that it is virtually impossible to tell if a person has an STD by just looking at him or her. There is only one sure way to prevent yourself from getting an STD—don't have sex; any kind of sex.

DO YOU KNOW THE FACTS?

Thirteen million people in the United States are affected by an STD each year.

Drugs and alcohol increase your chances of getting an STD, simply because of impaired judgment.

STDs occur most often in teenagers and young adults!

Having multiple partners increases your chance of being exposed to HIV or other STDs.

STDs can cause damage to major organs, like the heart, kidney, or even the brain, if it goes untreated.

There may be no symptoms with some STDs, but the disease can still be spread from person to person.[4]

But, just in case abstinence isn't the decision you make, there are a few things you need to know. First, there are ways to decrease your risks of developing an STD; things like condoms for example. If you make a choice to have sex, you *must* make a choice to protect yourself; so learn about condoms. A latex condom is the only method of birth control currently on the market that is effective in preventing the spread of HIV and STDs. That's because bacteria and viruses can't fit through the latex material. But remember, latex condoms could be affected by the way you store them and use them. If not used correctly, the condom may not be 100 percent effective, so keep that in mind. If you are sexually active or if you are considering becoming sexually active, you must have regular physical exams. Preventing STDs is the key! Remember it's a lot easier to prevent STDs than cure them.

Hold up. What about the risk of pregnancy? Some people think that just because they have diabetes they can't get pregnant or that they can't get a girl pregnant. Well, that's a bunch of bull. One thing that is true though, pregnancy can cause complications of diabetes to develop or get worse. Not only that, if the woman has poor diabetes control when she gets pregnant, there is an increased risk of birth defects for the baby. If poor glucose control continues throughout the pregnancy, the woman is at risk for complications like hypertension, premature labor, and even preterm delivery of the baby. The baby is also at risk if the mother's blood glucose level is not well controlled throughout the pregnancy. For example, when blood glucose levels are elevated in the mother, the baby packs on extra fat (the baby's insulin works just fine, so he or she gains extra weight from the extra glucose received through the placenta from the mom), leading to potential premature delivery. That's a problem because breathing difficulties can occur in the baby if his or her lungs are not well developed at birth. That's why it's really important to plan your pregnancy when you have diabetes, for your sake and the baby's sake as well.

As previously mentioned, when a woman has diabetes, she must strive for optimum blood glucose control *before* and *during* pregnancy; even *tighter* control than what she is used to in some circumstances. This requires diligent blood glucose monitoring, meal planning, exercise, and insulin/medication management. So, as you can probably already tell, you really need to have a good healthcare team in place before you begin to think about starting a family—to ensure a good outcome for everyone. And remember, there's more than your life at stake here; think through your decisions carefully. Some people think that decisions they make regarding their lives are justified because, after all, they are the only one affected by the decision. But the truth of the matter is, it is very rare that only one person is affected by a single decision, no matter what the subject matter is. See, there will always be someone in your life that will be affected by the decisions you make—whether it be your friends, your sisters or brothers, your parents, the people in your neighborhood or church or school, or even your community. Remember, no man is an island and every stone you toss leaves ripples in the water.

EATING DISORDERS—ANOREXIA AND BULIMIA

Maybe you've heard about these disorders before, maybe you haven't. They are eating disorders that can cause some people to lose their lives. So, without a doubt they are very serious. For some reason (scientists aren't really sure why, perhaps a chemical disorder in the brain or even stress from society to be thin) people with anorexia (usually women) starve themselves by eating very little. They seem to be obsessed about being thin and will do anything to prevent weight gain, no matter the cost. For some

Table 14.1. Don't be a casualty of unrealistic expectations. Remember: Magazine pictures are electronically edited and airbrushed! Looking like Barbie isn't physically possible!

	Average Woman	*Barbie*	*Store Mannequin*
Height	5'4"	6'0"	6'0"
Weight	145 lbs.	101 lbs.	Not available
Dress size	11–14	4	6
Bust	36–37"	39"	34"
Waist	29–31"	19"	23"
Hips	40–42"	33"	34"

*Anorexia Nervosa and Related Eating Disorders, Inc., (June 2002), "Statistics: How Many People Have Eating Disorders?" available at www.anred.com/stats.html (November 21, 2002).

THE SAD FACTS

One out of every hundred young women between ten and twenty are starving themselves, sometimes to death.

One in every hundred females between the ages of twelve and eighteen have anorexia.

Four out of a hundred college-aged women have bulimia.

Fifty percent of people who have been anorexic develop bulimia or bulimic patterns.

Without treatment, up to 20 percent of people with serious eating disorders die. With treatment, that number falls to 2–3 percent.[5]

reason, even if they are skeleton thin, they see themselves as being fat. This intense fear of being fat is what appears to drive them to starve. Starvation causes the body to slow down the natural body processes. For example, the blood pressure lowers and breathing becomes slower. Eventually the skin becomes dry, and hair and nails become brittle. Oftentimes the person will complain of feeling lightheaded, cold, and have constipation. If this situation is allowed to continue, the electrolytes in the body become so imbalanced that eventually the heart fails and the person dies.

Sometimes people with eating disorders will eat. Some, in fact, eat large amounts of food (bingeing) but then get rid of it by vomiting or by taking laxatives right away (purging). This is known as bulimia. Once people begin bingeing and purging, usually because they're on a diet, the situation can easily get out of control. Extreme purging changes the body's balance of sodium, potassium, and other electrolytes very quickly. This

---

FOR HELP WITH EATING DISORDERS . . .

Anorexia Nervosa and Bulimia Association (ANAB) Call (613) 547-3684

Eating Disorders Awareness and Prevention (EDAP) www.nationaleatingdisorders.org Call (800) 931-2237

The Center for Eating Disorders www.eating disorders.com Call (410) 427-2100

ANRED: Anorexia Nervosa and Related Eating Disorders www.anred.com Call (541) 344-1144

National Association of Anorexia Nervosa and Associated Disorders www.anad.org Call 847-831-3438

American Anorexia/Bulimia Association Call (212) 501-8351

Center for the Study of Anorexia and Bulimia Call (212) 333-3444, or write to 1841 Broadway, 4th Floor, New York, NY 10023

National Eating Disorders Organization Call (918) 481-4044, or write to 6655 South Yale Avenue, Tulsa, OK 74136

National Institute of Mental Health Eating Disorders Program Call (301) 496-1891, or write to Building 10, Room 35231, Bethesda, MD 20892

can cause the person to be very tired, have irregular heartbeats, and even have seizures! Repeated vomiting can damage the stomach and esophagus (the tube that carries food to the stomach) and damage the tooth enamel.

This is a very sad situation because most people find it difficult to stop their bulimic or anoretic behavior by themselves, yet they don't always seek professional help. And if they don't get help, the disorders can lead to severe health problems. See, many people with eating disorders don't feel as though they have much control over anything. By controlling their own bodies, people with eating disorders feel as though they can get back some control in their lives, even if it's unhealthy.

The good news is that there is help! There are medications that are currently being studied to help a person cope with the disorder, but like anything else, early treatment is the key. Besides medication, treatment may include therapy, nutrition counseling, behavior modification, or even self-help groups. Therapy can last a year or even more, but is usually on an outpatient basis, unless the person has life-threatening physical symptoms or severe psychological problems. If you think you have bulimia or anorexia, remember that you're not alone. This is a health problem that requires professional help.

NOTES

1. "Alcohol and Women," available at www.alb2c3.com/drugs/alc03.htm (November 3, 2002).

2. American Lung Association (June 2002), "American Lung Association Fact Sheet Smoking," available at www.lungusa.org/tobacco/smoking_factsheet99.html (July 26, 2002).

3. American Lung Association, "American Lung Association Fact Sheet Smoking."

4. National Institute of Allergy and Infectious Diseases (NIAID) and National Institutes of Health (NIH), "An Introduction to Sexually Transmitted Diseases," available at www.niaid.nih.gov/factsheets/stdinfo.htm (November 21, 2002).

5. Anorexia Nervosa and Related Eating Disorders, Inc., (June 2002), "Statistics: How Many People Have Eating Disorders?" available at www.anred.com/stats.html (November 21, 2002).

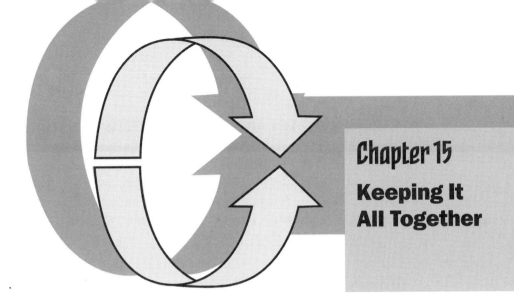

Chapter 15
Keeping It All Together

Granted, having diabetes is no walk in the park. But your life can and *will be* normal. Remember one thing, you are just like everyone else, you just happen to have diabetes. That's not to say that it's not difficult trying to keep up with the daily regime of diabetes self-management. In fact, sometimes it seems down right impossible! The hormonal changes that occur during adolescence and early adulthood can cause havoc on your blood glucose control. You probably feel like you're on a roller coaster and can't get off! That's because during this time in your life your body's normal epinephrine response to changes in blood glucose are greater than usual. To make matters even more complicated, there is also a potential for insulin resistance at this time due to hormonal changes. What that means is, the insulin that's in your body can't work as well as it should, while at the same time the body becomes more sensitive to epinephrine, causing the liver to dump more glucose in the blood. Even though this is difficult (really difficult), don't give up. This is not the time to be tempted to skip your regularly scheduled insulin doses, forget to take your oral diabetes medication, or give up on your meal plan. That can get you into some real serious trouble pretty quick!

What really helps is a trip to your healthcare practitioner. No one should be expected to go through this alone, and you are no exception! Get help from someone who can look at the situation objectively and give you some good sound advice.

DEALING WITH THE EMOTIONAL ROLLER COASTER!

It's true that the demands of diabetes management often come in conflict with the demands of everyday life. Diabetes is there 24/7—there's no diabetes vacation, no diabetes holiday, and no diabetes escape! To make matters worse, who likes getting stuck with a needle on a daily basis, or getting up to check blood glucose every morning without exception? Then as if someone were playing a cruel joke, all this work, all this time and commitment, yet all those stinking blood glucose levels are still all over the place! Give me a break! Who needs this crap!

Unfortunately, diabetes treatment is still not perfect, neither are the methods we currently have available to monitor the treatment. But, these treatments and tools keep people healthy during their entire lifetimes, albeit an unpleasant ritual. But keep in mind, as you get older and your hormones become more regulated, it should be easier to control your blood sugar again. Until that time we need to talk about how to keep from feeling overwhelmed or even depressed when you're weighed down with daily life.

Depression seems to be more common in people with diabetes than it is in the general population. Some statistics indicate 25–40 percent of those who have diabetes suffer from symptoms of depression.[1] Not only that, but depression can then lead to apathy in people with diabetes. That just means they don't care about doing anything to stay healthy anymore. As a result, they exercise less, eat more, and end up with high blood glucose levels. For some reason females tend to be affected more than males.[2] But again, the key is prevention! There are things you can do to prevent this from ever happening.

First, start by recognizing the symptoms and where these symptoms come from. Just recognizing typical feelings and behaviors of people your own age is a great starting point. See, even if you didn't have diabetes you would likely be experiencing some feelings of frustration from time to time, just because of where you are in your life! For example, some teens struggle with their self-esteem as they search for their own identity. Changes in your body and the desire for acceptance make it difficult to decide whether you are *normal*. Well relax; you are very normal!

Sometimes the media make the situation even more problematic by bombarding television and movies with advertisements of picture-perfect people! Who wouldn't be affected by that day after day? For one thing, women weren't made to be that skinny. Second of all, men don't naturally have that much muscle either! It's important for you to realize that your self-worth shouldn't be measured against external variables. You're much better off measuring yourself against a measuring stick that's designed especially for you! Or even better, focus on what's really important, which is to lead a healthy lifestyle. In addition, figure out what makes you happy. Knowing what makes you happy and how to meet your goals can make you feel capable, strong, and in control of your life. A positive attitude and a healthy lifestyle are a great combination. That's much better than trying to fit into an unrealistic world. That only leads to problems, like drinking and drugs. People turn to these ineffective coping mechanisms when they feel like they can't take it any more, and they think drugs will help. But in reality that really sends them spiraling.

SO, WHAT CAN YOU DO?

You need to start looking at yourself and your situation through new eyes! If you look at your diabetes through new eyes you'll be able to see more effective ways of coping with the disease. That way you'll never get to the point where you're overwhelmed. See, if you learn to cope with what life deals you, you're more apt to care for your diabetes effectively, instead of just saying "to heck with it" and throwing in the towel one day. The next time you're hearing negative comments coming from within, tell yourself to stop. Instead, try replacing those thoughts with something positive. Do this *every* time, *every* day. By focusing on the good things you do and the positive aspects of your life, you can change how you feel about yourself and your diabetes.

> I have always just told my friends I have diabetes and they accept me for me! —Nikki

WHAT IF I NEED SOMEONE TO HELP ME?

Some teens with diabetes decide not to tell their friends that they have diabetes because they don't want to be treated differently, or because they just don't want to feel different. While it's normal to experience these types of feelings and emotions, sometimes these low feelings start and they don't ever seem to go away. Sometimes persistent low feelings are too much to handle alone. You may even be afraid to tell your friends how you're feeling. At this point it is easy to slip into depression and lose interest in activities or friends. If this happens to you, the best thing for you to do is to talk to someone, anyone that you trust and have an open relationship with. You may want to ask your healthcare practitioner about getting some additional support, especially if you're having trouble dealing with having diabetes at school, at home, or with friends.

EMOTIONAL PERSPECTIVE

Having someone to talk to can help you put your feelings into perspective. Not only that, but when you feel better emotionally, it's likely that your blood glucose level will reflect that positive change. Yes, even your emotions can affect your blood glucose level! So, the most important thing to remember is to get help if you feel like your thoughts or emotions are affecting your life. We're not talking about the day-to-day feelings of everyday life; it's more the long-term feeling of sadness that gets in the way of living.

Some symptoms of depression may include feeling really tired, having trouble sleeping, eating everything and anything, or maybe nothing sparks your appetite anymore. Some people don't feel like doing anything because nothing sounds like fun. Don't forget that there are thousands of teens out there just like you! They're facing the same challenges and frustrations. So

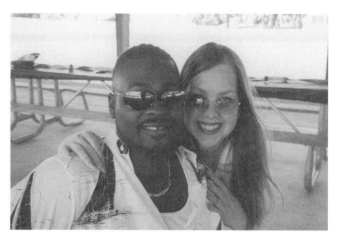

you're not alone! You just need time to learn how to handle these challenges in the most healthful way! Another thing, don't be afraid to get involved in your local support group. Support groups are great because you get to meet other people your same age that might be able to give you some tips on what has worked for them! For example, maybe there's one thing, that really bothers you about your diabetes or diabetes management. Well, if you talk with someone who's going through the same thing, you might be surprised to find out that they've already worked through the very same situation and may have some practical advice to get you through it!

NOTES

1. Richard Rubin, "Diabetes Overwhelmus: Diagnosis, Causes and Treatment," *Practical Diabetology* 19, no. 4 (2000): 30.

2. William H. Polonsky and Christopher G. Parkin, "Depression in Patients with Diabetes: Seven Facts Every Health-Care Provider Should Know," *Practical Diabetology* 20, no. 4 (2001): 21.

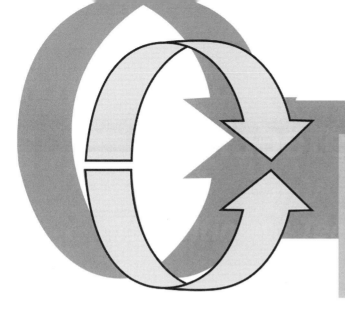

Chapter 16

The Real Deal behind the Wheel!

Finally! You're behind the wheel of your red Mustang convertible, tooling down the open highway with the wind in your hair. You can feel the warmth of the sun on your arms and smell the ocean in the air! Ah, freedom—this is livin'! Every teenager's dream right? Yeah, life is good! Even if your first car doesn't exactly live up to your *dream car*, there's nothing like being able to jump behind the wheel, turn up the radio, crank the windows down, and open it up on the neighborhood highway (obeying speed limits at all times, of course). Well, the goal of this chapter is to give you some good sound advice that will help you maintain that *privilege* through your golden years.

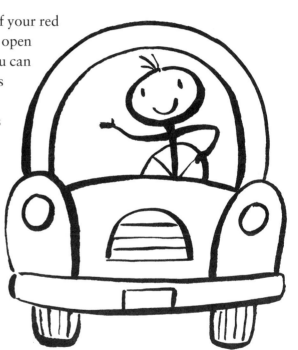

DRIVING'S A PRIVILEGE?

Yeah, driving really is a privilege. You probably already know that because you've had to jump through all kinds of hoops just to get your driver's license to begin with right? Okay, so what do you have to know to *keep* the license you've worked so hard for? Glad you asked! First of all, just like everything else we've discussed so far, the key is prevention. In this case, we're talking about preventing low blood glucose while driving. See, the stats on this are really scary. Even though the research on this subject is old and not very rigorous, there is still enough concern regarding the results to get your attention. For example, back in 1989 this group published an article that looked at people with diabetes (taking insulin) who drive. The results indicated that up to one-third of the people with diabetes that were surveyed had experienced hypoglycemia (low blood glucose) symptoms while driving.[1] Another group reported that 34 percent of the people they looked at with diabetes had experienced *severe* hypoglycemia (loss of consciousness or couldn't treat themselves) while driving during the previous six months.[2] Boy, if that's not a wakeup call, what is?

THAT WON'T HAPPEN TO ME! I KNOW WHEN I'M LOW!

If you're thinking to yourself, "That won't happen to me," well, hope you're right. But just in case, make sure you check your blood glucose *before* you get behind the wheel! There's still some more research out there you should know about.

**I always check my blood glucose before I drive.
—Nikki**

The research indicates that even mild hypoglycemia (60–65 mg/dl) can impair cognitive-motor function. What that means is your reaction time will be slower, your attention and concentration will be disrupted, even your ability to problem solve and make decisions will be impaired. So what does all that mean? Well, let's take a look at some of the research that has been done that looked at the relationship between blood glucose level and driving skills. These studies used a driving simulator, so no one would get hurt! They showed that driving skills got worse as the blood glucose level dropped between 67 and 45 mg/dl.[3] Okay, no big surprise, right? If the blood glucose level is low, the brain function starts to decline as well. But, here's the kicker, even though these people knew they had stuff in the car simulator to treat low blood glucose, and were instructed to go ahead and treat themselves if they were feeling low, only 32 percent attempted to treat their symptoms during the driving scenario! Wow! That's incredible; even though they felt low, most people did not treat their symptoms! What's even more incredible is that when tested further, about 40–45 percent of the time people said they *would* drive even when they estimated their blood glucose between 60 and 70 mg/dl.[4] And they said they would drive 18 to 38 percent of the time when they estimated their blood glucose to be less than 40 mg/dl!! Makes you want to stay off the road doesn't it?

WHAT CAN YOU DO TO PREVENT HYPOGLYCEMIA WHILE DRIVING?

There are a few simple steps you can take to make sure you stay safe while driving. First, *always* check your blood glucose level before you get into the car to drive. Don't just guess at what your blood glucose level is, you can't afford to take the chance on being wrong! Also, if your blood glucose is mildly low (60–65 mg/dl), treat yourself first, before you get behind the wheel. Which brings us to another very good point: make sure you keep 15 grams of carbohydrate in your car at all times. You never know when you'll need it. And another thing, don't skip meals and drive, that's not safe. Believe it or not there have been a few people that have actually done that. This one particular guy got up in the morning with an elevated blood glucose level, so he took his insulin just like he normally would. Then he decided he would go out to eat breakfast. So he got in his car and drove to the restaurant. Well, needless to say this guy didn't make it to the restaurant; he had an accident on the way. Luckily he didn't kill himself or anyone else. But not everyone is that lucky. Above all, if you are already driving and you start to feel low, pull off the road, eat 15 grams of carbohydrates, and wait fifteen minutes to see if your blood glucose level returns to a safe level for driving. A good target is at least 80 mg/dl before you start to drive. Remember, driving is a privilege, and that privilege can be removed if safety measures aren't followed. For example, did you know that in some states if you have a seizure related to severe hypoglycemia you must wait six months without having another seizure before you can drive again? So, the key here is prevention. Play it safe; you'll be happy you did in the long run.

DREAMING ABOUT DRIVING

Nikki had a dream just after she got her driver's license. She said it was the weirdest dream because it seemed so real. Ever have those kinds of dreams? Well, anyway in her dream she was driving down the road near home, when she noticed a police car behind her with the flashers on. She panicked of course, but immediately pulled over. Well, the officer came over to her car window and told her that she was driving erratically and wanted to know if she had been drinking. She was shocked that he had asked her that and snapped back, "No!" Well, that was all it took, the police officer asked her to get out of the car and for permission to search the vehicle. She gave him permission, then immediately began crying hysterically.

The officer, unaffected by her crying, proceeded to search her vehicle. He opened her glove box (seems like a likely place to start) and was startled when

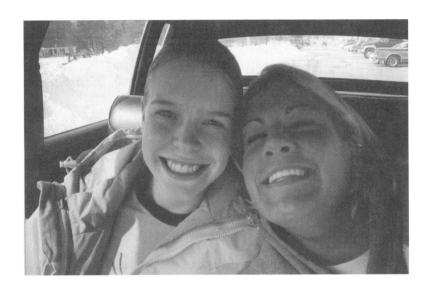

thousands of unwrapped glucose tablets came flying out of the glove compartment. This sent Nikki into a tailspin. The officer asked for an explanation, but Nikki couldn't figure out what the tablets were, because her blood glucose level was so low! She just couldn't think! So the officer continued searching the car. He moved to the front of the vehicle,

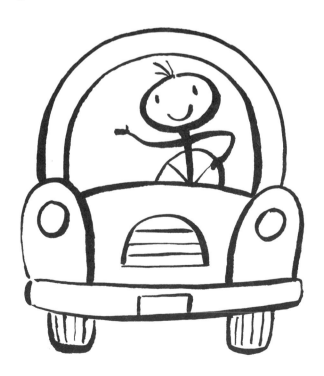

RULES OF THE ROAD TO LIVE BY

- Check your blood glucose level before driving—every time!
- Treat hypoglycemia before driving, then wait until your blood glucose level is 80 mg/dl before driving.
- Make sure that you have 15 grams of carbohydrates in your car at all times (glucose tablets work great).
- If you feel low, pull off the road, check your blood glucose level, treat low blood glucose, wait 15 minutes until your blood glucose level returns to 80 mg/dl.

popped the hood and to his surprise (and Nikki's) there were hundreds of blood glucose monitors on top of the motor! Just sitting there! Luckily, the alarm went off and Nikki woke up, realizing that it had all been a dream. But she understood from her dream how important it is to have some form of diabetes identification on you at all times, just in case *you* have to explain some unusual circumstances to a police officer, when it isn't a dream!

NOTES

1. Steven A., M. Roberts, R. McKane, A. Atkinson, P. Bell, and J. Hayes, "Motor Vehicle Driving Among Diabetics Taking Insulin and Non-Diabetics," *British Medical Journal* 299, (1989): 591–95.

2. Frier B., D. Matthews, J. Steele, L. Duncan, "Driving and Insulin-Dependent Diabetes," *Lancet* 1 (1980): 1232–34.

3. Daniel J. Cox, Linda A. Gonder-Frederick, and William L. Clarke, "Driving Decrements in Type 1 Diabetes During Moderate Hypoglycemia," *Diabetes* 42, (1993): 239–43.

4. William L. Clarke, Daniel J. Cox, Linda A. Gonder-Frederick, and Boris Kovatchev, "Hypoglycemia and the Decision to Drive a Motor Vehicle by Persons with Diabetes," *Journal of the American Medical Association* 282 (1999): 750–54.

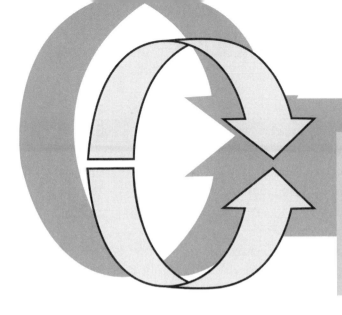

Today is the day! Yeah! Traveling off to the far ends of the earth to explore unchartered lands. No one but you, fresh ocean breezes, and wide-open spaces! You've waited a long time for this trip and you've planned every detail! Now you want things to go right; this is your time. Time you well deserve. Traveling is good for the mind, soul, and spirit. It opens your eyes to different cultures and allows you to grow as a person. By all means, take advantage of every opportunity in life. Whatever you do, don't let your diabetes be the reason you miss out on the trip of a lifetime!

What? You say diabetes *has* gotten in your way? You can't travel because it's too much of a hassle to lug around all that stuff to manage your disease, or maybe you feel like you can't travel because you're afraid customs officers won't allow you to enter the country with all that paraphernalia? Nonsense! You can go anywhere your heart desires, with a little preparation!

Just like *everything* else we've discussed so far, anything is possible,

Bon Voyage!

given the proper tools and opportunity! Let's discuss what it takes to be a world traveler. To begin, make sure you plan ahead. Get yourself an appointment with your healthcare practitioner several months before your trip. That way you'll be

159

sure to have all the necessary paperwork and vaccinations taken care of ahead of time. It's a good idea to get a letter from your physician (on his/her letterhead) that states you have diabetes and how you manage the disease. This letter will help you in the event there is ever any question regarding why you are carrying all your medical supplies.

Speaking of medical supplies, the key here is to bring enough supplies for the time you'll be gone plus another couple of weeks, just in case you are detained. The just in case strategy always works! Now, let's say you're going to be gone for two weeks. You're using an insulin pump to manage your diabetes and you just recently changed the pump batteries. Should you bring extra batteries for the pump, even though you just changed them and they *should* last for at least several more months? Yes, yes, yes!! Remember, prevention is the key. You never know when something strange will happen and then there you'll be, in the middle of nowhere, without any batteries or any way of getting batteries. So prepare for the unexpected!

Which brings up a good point. Where should you put all of this stuff? Perhaps you should pack it in your checked luggage? After all you did bring a lot of extra stuff, which takes up a lot of room. No, no, no!! This is really important. Carry all those extra supplies *with* you! Yes, put the supplies in a carry-on bag and keep them with you at all times. Again, this is the only way you can be sure that you'll have all of the supplies you'll need for your trip. See, if you put this stuff in your luggage, then check the luggage for the flight, what happens if your luggage is lost? Not a good situation, right? So, be prepared and keep it with you.

Now, the other thing to remember is that you should also keep your insulin bottles and/or oral medication with you. And bring the original insulin box with the prescription label on it; this will save you extra time when going through security checkpoints. Bringing extra bottles of insulin along just in case is also a good idea, and carry them with you. Here again, if you were to pack the insulin in a suitcase and check it in, you have no way of knowing what happens to that suitcase from the time you leave until the time you arrive at your destination. That's important to consider because the storage compartments on planes are *not* temperature regulated. So, it is possible that you could be exposing your insulin to temperatures of 125° F or −20° F, and you wouldn't know the difference; until of course you went to use your insulin and it was discolored or had particles in it. Worse yet, what if the insulin looked the same and you used it? Certainly afterward you would figure out that something was wrong when your blood glucose level suddenly skyrocketed! Oh, another thing to consider regarding your insulin or oral medication, you may be traveling to a country that may not carry the same insulin concentration or oral medication that you take. For example, in some countries insulin is distributed in U-80 concentration instead of the U-100 that is used in the United States. Not only that, the syringes in those countries are also made specifically for use with U-80 insulin. So see, planning ahead can really prevent a whole lot of headaches down the road!

WHAT DO YOU NEED TO BRING WHEN YOU'RE TRAVELING?

You may be wondering what you need to bring along with you when traveling. Well, as mentioned previously, you need to take the supplies that you'll need for the time that you're gone plus some extra for *just in case*. You'll also need those extra supplies for monitoring as well. See, when you're traveling you really need to pay close attention to your blood glucose level. That means extra tests for sure. Once again, remember to bring extra

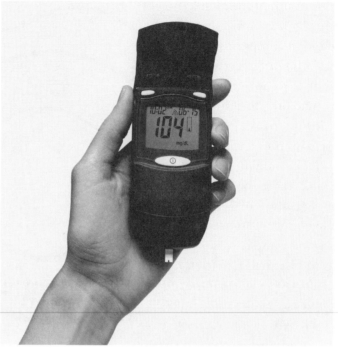

Compact meter courtesy of Roche Diagnostics

batteries for the glucose monitor, and even bring an extra glucose monitor if you have one. You don't want to jeopardize your trip because of a glucose monitor that suddenly stops working.

If you use an insulin pump, you'll need to bring all the supplies for your pump, tube changes, and of course extra batteries and insulin. Notify security screeners that you are wearing an insulin pump and show them, rather than removing it from your body. You'll also need to bring some traditional syringes, in the event that something happens to your pump while you're gone. That way you'll be able to give yourself insulin with a syringe until you are able to get the problem resolved. Certainly you've heard all this stuff before, but it's worth repeating.

It doesn't hurt to bring along a glucagon kit as well (used to treat severe hypoglycemia when you are unable to take anything by mouth). But, what's equally important is having someone available who knows how to use it! It won't do you any good to have glucagon in your bag if no one knows it's in there or if no one knows how to use it. On that same note, bring 15 grams of carbohydrates along as well to treat low blood glucose levels. Glucose tablets work really well because they're easy to carry and don't take up a lot of space. It also helps if you can fit some type of carbohydrate-containing snacks and maybe even some bottled water in your carry-on bag, too. That way if the only thing they're serving on the plane is pretzels, you'll have a back up! If you are fortunate enough to have the option of an in-flight meal, it really isn't necessary to order a diabetic meal. Most people prefer to order a regular meal and adjust their insulin based on the carbohydrate content.

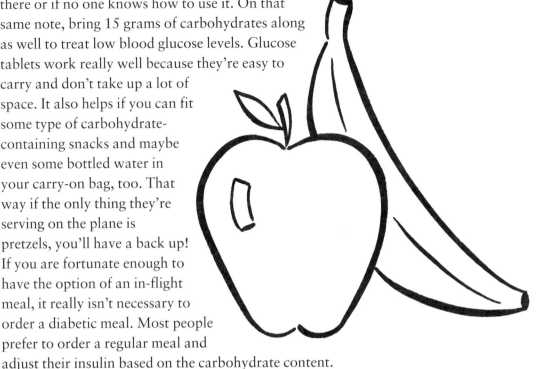

Oh, you'll also want to bring medications for traveler's diarrhea, nausea and vomiting, headaches, and so forth based on what your physician recommends. And don't be afraid to get up and walk around when you're on a long flight. It really helps your circulation; it's a good practice for anyone!

WHAT ABOUT CROSSING TIME ZONES?

It sure can be confusing when you're traveling across time zones. Travelers always ask, "When should I take my insulin?" "How should I change my eating patterns?" Well again, the best way to deal with this situation is to plan ahead. Ask your healthcare practitioner what he or she recommends. But, just to give you an example, if you are traveling east, you will lose time out of the day. On the other hand, if you are traveling west, you will gain time in the day. So having said that, if you lose time in the day, it just makes sense that you will need to cut back on your intermediate acting insulin (background insulin) to prevent low blood glucose. If you're a pump user, the same holds true for you. You'll need to make

163

QUICK TIPS FOR TRAVELING WITH DIABETES

- See your physician several months/weeks before your trip—get a letter indicating that you have diabetes.
- Get any necessary vaccines.
- Bring extra supplies.
- Bring extra insulin.
- Bring glucagon.
- Bring 15 grams of carbohydrates to treat low blood glucose.
- Wear diabetes identification.
- Pack carbohydrate-containing snacks and bottled water for the trip.
- Take comfortable shoes.
- Don't go barefoot!
- Don't eat it if it's not cooked and don't drink it if it's not bottled!
- Monitor your blood glucose frequently!

Have Fun!!

adjustments in your basal rates. The adjustments you'll need to make depend on what you and your healthcare practitioner come up with. Some clinics tell their patients to cut back on the dose by whatever the percentage of twenty-four hours is lost.[1] On the other hand, if you are adding hours to the day, injections of your fast or rapid acting insulin, which is given before meals, can be added every four to six hours to cover the extra time.[2] Generally speaking, if you don't gain or lose more than three hours in a day, then no change in insulin is needed. If you are taking oral medication to manage your diabetes, you may need to make changes in your treatment plan as well. However, that will depend on what you are taking. So, no matter what you use to manage your diabetes, remember to check with your healthcare professional to work out a plan before you leave! And remember, with all these changes going on it's going to be real important for you to monitor your blood glucose level frequently. How else will you know if what you've changed is working?

As far as changing your eating patterns are concerned, the same information applies. You may need an extra meal or snack if you are traveling west. Plan ahead for this! Bring extra snacks for long trips and stay on home time during travel. Then, change your watch to current time when you get to your travel destination.

Now when you get there, remember that the food and water may be different from that at home. So, your body may protest if you indulge without proper precaution.

- ◎ **Rule number 1—Don't drink the water in underdeveloped countries. And remember ice is made from water!**
- ◎ **Rule number 2—Don't eat anything raw! That goes for fruits and vegetables as well.**
- ◎ **Rule number 3—Remember to bring comfortable clothes and shoes that fit well. You'll probably be doing a lot of walking, so take care of your feet! Remember, never go barefoot! Your feet take you where you're going, so take care of them!**

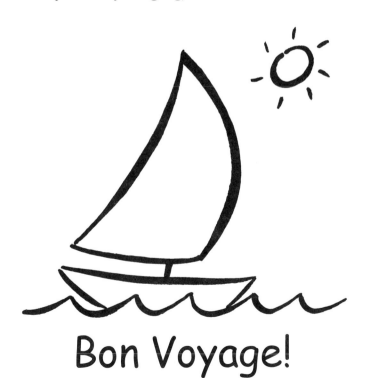

Bon Voyage!

NOTES

1. Martha M. Funnell, Cheryl Hunt, Karmeen Kulkarni, Richard R. Rubin, and Peggy C. Yarborough, *A Core Curriculum for Diabetes Education* (Chicago: American Association of Diabetes Educators, 1998), 220.

2. Funnell et al., *A Core Curriculum for Diabetes Education*, 221.

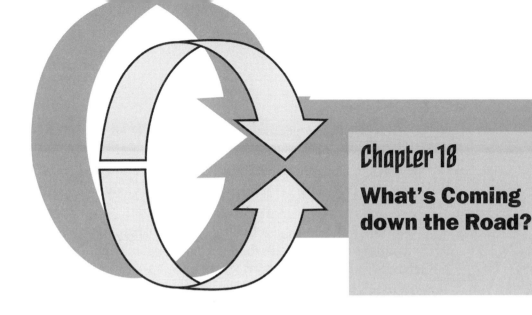

Chapter 18
What's Coming down the Road?

There is certainly a need for basic research to find solutions to key challenges in the development, management, and ultimately the cure for diabetes. These challenges are being investigated on the global front, which is great for people with diabetes. It will certainly take a collaborative effort within the global diabetes community to bridge the gap between what we know now and what we need to know to effectively eliminate this disease. So, if you've ever thought to yourself, "They can put a man on the moon, why can't they come up with something to cure diabetes?" rest assured there are literally teams of scientists working diligently to come up with the cure for diabetes.

WHAT'S CURRENTLY BEING INVESTIGATED: DIABETES RESEARCH?

Until a cure is found, we can focus our thoughts on those accomplishments already made in the field of diabetes research. For example, we are fortunate that there have been big breakthroughs in the management of diabetes and ways in which a person with diabetes can prevent or delay the onset of complications. Yes, we have certainly come a long way since 1921 when Drs. Banting and Best from Toronto, Canada, discovered insulin. At that time, remember, it was thought that insulin was the cure for diabetes. Soon afterward, though, they discovered that insulin was not a cure, rather a means of keeping a person alive. It was only after people lived for years with diabetes that scientists discovered there were complications that developed if blood glucose levels remained elevated. So you see, there have been big advancements in the field of diabetes research to be happy about. Our job now is to advocate for research to continue in this very important area and to support organizations that have made diabetes a priority.

Beta cell transplant is a hot topic in the diabetes research community today. What's that? Well, if you remember, beta cells are the cells located in the islets of Langerhans (the tail of the pancreas) that are responsible for making the hormone insulin. When type 1 diabetes develops, those cells are destroyed by the immune system; they can no longer produce any insulin. As a result, the person's blood glucose level remains high because the glucose has no way of getting into the cells.

Okay, so what happens with a beta cell transplant? Good question! Healthy beta cells are transplanted into the person with type 1 diabetes (into the liver through a needle) in hopes that the cells will respond the way the islet cells respond in a healthy pancreas. The beta cell transplant process, known as the Edmonton Protocol, is currently being trialed at the University of Alberta in Edmonton, Canada. What they have found is that this indeed is the case, if the cells can be protected from the immune system (in other words, not destroyed again). Currently, the only known way to prevent the transplanted beta

---

ROSALYN YALOW, PHD

◎ Discovered how to measure insulin precisely, which won her the Nobel Prize in Physiology and Medicine in 1977.

◎ Because Dr. Yalow and her colleagues discovered a way to measure insulin in the blood, they were able to identify that people with type 1 diabetes had very low (if any) amounts of insulin available. At the same time when they looked at people with type 2 diabetes they found something very different. These people had high levels of insulin in the blood (it just wasn't working). This is what really proved that there were indeed different types of diabetes.

◎ Her work helped lead the way to more effective diagnosis and treatment of diabetes and other diseases.[1]

cells from being attacked by the immune system is to give the person anti-rejection medications for the rest of his or her life. Unfortunately, these drugs can lead to infection and certain kinds of cancers. Because of these risks (even though they are small), the research on beta cell transplants has only been done on those individuals who are having a hard time maintaining control with insulin, having real bad lows, having wide variations in blood glucose levels, or even those people who are developing complications from diabetes. So you can see it's really not for the general public with diabetes. They really have to weigh out the benefits versus the risks right now.

However, there are other areas of promise currently being researched as well. Scientists in the United States and Belgium are looking at how they can stop the body from destroying the beta cells when type 1 diabetes is first developing. They are doing this by giving people an antibody early after diagnosis (within six weeks) to see if it will stop the body from destroying the beta cells. So let's say you are just diagnosed with diabetes, they give you these antibodies that stop the body from destroying the remainder of the beta cells. The only problem is, there are only a few beta cells left, certainly not enough to maintain normal blood glucose levels. So, now what? Well, that's where another study comes in to play. This study is looking at how to get beta cells to reproduce within the body of a person with diabetes. In other words, scientists are trying to figure out a way they can get the beta cells that are left to reproduce and make more functioning beta cells!

THE UNITED STATES POSTAL SERVICE POSTAGE STAMP ABOUT DIABETES AWARENESS

- Released on March 16, 2001.
- Designed by artist James Steinberg.
- Includes two elements associated with diabetes testing and research—a microscope and a test tube containing blood.
- The design communicates the importance of diabetes awareness and early detection.

There are even studies out there right now that are looking at trying to predict who is more likely to develop diabetes. For example, genetics trials are trying to isolate the markers that indicate a person will develop diabetes so they can do something to either prevent it from happening or slow down the onset.

Speaking of identifying those people at high risk for diabetes, one of the most significant recent research trials was the Diabetes Prevention Trial—Type 1. It was made up of two parts: one part looked at whether giving people at 50 percent risk of developing diabetes an injection of insulin daily over time would prevent the disease; the second part looked at whether giving people who were at 25–50 percent risk of developing diabetes oral insulin to prevent the disease. As it turned out the insulin injections had no effect on delaying the onset of diabetes; however, the oral insulin part of the study is still ongoing. Because of this research there are now new immunosuppressive agents (drugs that suppress the immune system) being studied in new-onset type 1 patients. Anyway you look at it, current research is pretty exciting!

WHO ARE THE BIG PLAYERS IN DIABETES RESEARCH?

As mentioned previously, diabetes research is currently a global project. There are multiple players involved in this search for a cure and for a better life for people who have diabetes. There are projects that are currently being investigated in Alberta, Canada, where the concept of beta cell transplant was realized and developed into a protocol. In 1999, TrialNet was developed to help support trials in diabetes research. The National Institute of Health, the National Institute for Diabetes, Digestive and Kidney Diseases, the National Institute of Allergy and Infectious Diseases, and the National Institute of Child Health and Human Development support this organization. TrialNet was actually developed as a result of the work that was being done in the Diabetes Prevention Trial—Type 1.

The Immune Tolerance Network is another example of a group of institutions that are working together to fund research in the area of transplant and immune tolerance strategies. The

Juvenile Diabetes Research Foundation, the National Institute for Diabetes, Digestive and Kidney Disease, and the National Institute of Allergy and Infectious Diseases support this group and the beta cell transplantation trial they are currently embarking on in nine areas of the United States.

In addition, in 2002 the Juvenile Diabetes Research Foundation Center for Beta Cell Therapy was established in Europe. The goal of this center is to intensify the search for a cure, as well as develop solutions to restoring normal blood glucose levels in people with type 1 diabetes. Another area to look for new research is Paris, France. At Inserm, which is the National Institute of Health and Medical Research in France, they are trying to get precursor cells (these are cells that haven't developed into specific cells yet) to develop into insulin-producing cells. Also, in Denmark, at the Hagedorn Research Laboratory, researchers are trying to develop ways to increase the amount of human beta cells that are available for transplant. And finally, in Sweden the Swedish Research Council and the Swedish Diabetes Association Research Foundation are looking at the role of stem cells in curing type 1 diabetes.

ADVANCEMENTS IN DIABETES MANAGEMENT

In addition to the work that is being done to find a cure or to prevent the onset of diabetes, there is also a lot being done to help make the lives of people with diabetes better. For example, you've probably heard about the glucose monitor on the market that doesn't require repeated blood glucose samples. Cignus is the company that developed this product. The monitor is able to check your blood glucose through the fluid in your skin for periods up to twelve hours. However, you do have to calibrate the monitor against a traditional blood glucose monitor whenever you change the sensing pad (approximately every twelve hours). In addition to this nontraditional glucose monitor, there are a variety of alternative site testing glucose monitors now on the market. These monitors allow you to use your forearm or thigh for example, to check your blood glucose. They require a very small sample of blood, which allows the machine to be used on areas that weren't available for testing previously.

If you have an interest in trying one of these monitors, call your certified diabetes educator for more information.

Are you the kind of person who just cringes when you see a needle? Boy, being diagnosed with diabetes really has been a struggle, hasn't it? Well, you'll be happy to know there are needleless injectors that are available to give insulin now instead of the traditional syringe. These devices use pressurized air to move the insulin through the skin into the fat tissue. If that doesn't sound any better, how about trying any of the needle injectors that are available. They use the same syringe, but the device is spring-loaded so the needle is inserted quickly. And the device hides the needle so you can't see it!

If you've decided to try pumping insulin, you'll be glad to hear there are many new pumps on the market! Several of these pumps have all the bells and whistles, but are small enough to hide in the most discrete places! Isn't it great that researchers and designers are continuously searching for a better product to assist you in your diabetes management?

Speaking of new insulin products, research scientists have been working on new methods for insulin delivery that don't involve needles. For example, there is insulin in the form of an oral inhaler that is currently in clinical trials. This method of delivery appears to have the same effectiveness as injected insulin, but offers the person with diabetes a mode of delivery that is more welcome to some. However, more research is necessary to see what, if any, side effects there are. So, it may be a while before we see this on the market.

Your Future Is Bright!

Certainly there are many other things currently being investigated in the field of diabetes as it relates to management, treatment, and even a cure for diabetes that we have not discussed here. What we have discussed was really meant to give you a glimpse of what is on the horizon—as well as hope for the future.

It Is My Dream . . .

It is my dream to be free from the worries of diabetes;
to have all children enjoy their candy from Halloween.
It is my dream that offers less worry and finger bruises.
A dream that I can stay up all night with my friends, and not
see the face from the ambulance driver in the morning from
having low blood sugar.

It is my dream that they will find a cure;
A cure that allows all those with diabetes to feel the
cool breeze of freedom come about them.
A cure that allows them to rejoice in their new feelings of life.

It is my dream that with a cure, life will be easier.
A cure would bring happiness
and joy to everyone's hearts.

It is my dream to battle against diabetes.
A dream to stand up strong
and control the inside of my body.

It is my dream that when I have reached the end of this battle, I
will stop and wonder, "How did I do this?"
But, I will know that I did, and that I did it well.
It is my dream that I awake with the sunlight shining in my
eyes, telling me it's time to start over.

It is my dream that is not so far in the future.
A dream that would be so wonderful,
so wonderful indeed.

This is my dream . . .

—*Nicole, age 17*
diagnosed with type 1 diabetes at age 3

NOTE

1. Sheldon H. Gottlieb, "Rosalyn Yalow: Diabetes and the Nobel Prize," *Diabetes Forecast* 55, no. 11 (2002): 31–33.

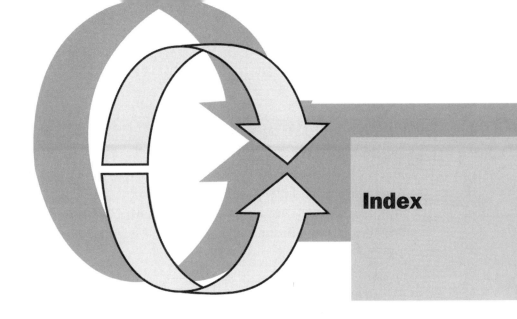

Index

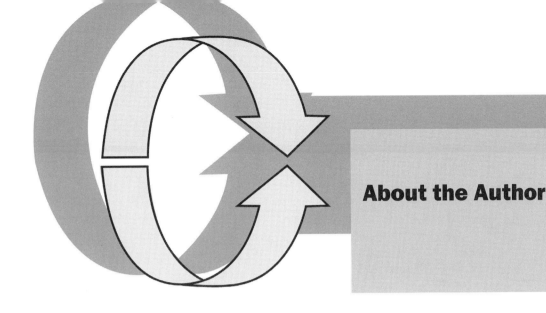

About the Author

Katherine Moran, MSN, RN, CDE received her master's degree in nursing from the University of Phoenix and is a certified diabetes educator. She is currently the clinical manager for the diabetes education program at St. John Hospital and Medical Center in Detroit, Michigan. She is also responsible for the system coordination of three additional St. John Health diabetes education programs located in urban, suburban, and rural areas northeast of Detroit. Kathy devoted her professional life to the education of those with diabetes after the diagnosis of her daughter, Nicole, with type 1 diabetes at age three.

She has extensive experience in educating people with diabetes, as well as healthcare professionals who care for the person with diabetes. Kathy has been a national presenter for the American Association of Diabetes Educators, Aventis Pharmaceutical, and for numerous professional and community seminars across the state of Michigan. Her most recent endeavors include co-authoring a manuscript titled "Diabetes Management in the School Setting: A Tool Kit" and a research project that utilized the tool kit to provide diabetes education for teachers and other school personnel in the school setting.

Kathy is also an advocate for people with diabetes. She sits on the American Diabetes Association's Government Relations Committee, Diabetes in the School task force, and has testified for diabetes issues in front of the Michigan Senate and House of Representatives.